Integrated Contraceptive and Sexual Healthcare

A practical guide

Sarah Bekaert
Development Nurse
City and Hackney Young People's Services

and

Alison White
Development Nurse
City and Hackney Young People's Services

Forewords by

Kathy French
Sexual Health Adviser
Royal College of Nursing

and

Kevin Miles
Nurse Consultant in Sexual Health
Camden Primary Care Trust

Radcliffe Publishing
Oxford • Seattle

Radcliffe Publishing Ltd
18 Marcham Road
Abingdon
Oxon OX14 1AA
United Kingdom

www.radcliffe-oxford.com
Electronic catalogue and worldwide online ordering facility.

New research and clinical experience can result in changes in treatment and drug therapy. Readers of this book should therefore check the most recent product information on any drug they may prescribe to ensure they are complying with the manufacturer's recommendations concerning dosage, the method and duration of administration, and contraindications. Neither the publisher nor the authors accept liability for any injury or damage arising from this publication.

British Library Cataloguing in Publication Data

A catalogue record for this book is available from the British Library.

ISBN-10: 1 85775 723 8
ISBN-13: 978 1 85775 723 1

Typeset by Aarontype Ltd, Easton, Bristol
Printed and bound by Alden (Malaysia)

Contents

Foreword

Sexual health has been seen as a key priority in the White Paper *Choosing Health* (2005) and this timely publication will go a long way in helping the many professionals in the field to deliver care as part of a team. For too long the speciality of sexual health has been divided in terms of service provision but also in the delivery of publications.

With the integration of many sexual health services, this well laid out book will help practitioners new to the field of sexual health navigate their way through the many aspects of care, providing them with useful references and websites.

Nurses within this speciality are clearly taking a lead in providing services which the clients value, and are able to use their knowledge and skills to function in a way unthinkable 10 years ago. Nurses have the day-to-day experience of working in the field and producing such a book will inspire others to follow.

I am delighted with the publication of this book for nurses and others and I am sure the educators will consider this publication essential reading for pre- and post-registration students in sexual health.

Kathy French
Sexual Health Adviser
Royal College of Nursing
April 2006

Foreword

Sexually transmitted infections (STIs) continue to be reported in increasing numbers across the United Kingdom; the consequences of which are now being taken seriously by political leaders. In 2001 the National Strategy for Sexual Health and HIV placed the provision of services for STIs, HIV and contraception firmly on the public health agenda. Sexual health is now a top priority for the NHS with four Public Service Agreement (PSA) targets aiming to: i) reduce teenage pregnancy; ii) reduce the incidence of gonorrhoea; iii) increase access to genitourinary medicine (GUM) services within 48 hours, and; iv) increase the number of people aged 15 to 24 accepting chlamydia screeening.

Several issues have repeatedly emerged in a number of the government's policy directives, namely, the concept of integrated contraceptive and sexual healthcare, commonly referred to as 'one-stop-shop' models of care, and the expanding role that nurses in the modern NHS have to play. Nurses are now undertaking more advanced practice roles and are increasingly becoming the first-line providers of care for people presenting with concerns about contraception and sexual health. Traditionally this has been through 'vertical' models of care; clients needing STI screening would go to a GUM clinic and those requiring contraception to a family planning service. However, nurses are now challenging the traditions of contraceptive and sexual healthcare to provide integrated models that are more aligned with the needs of the population that they serve.

As such, the knowledge and skills that nurses now require in both contraceptive and sexual healthcare are essential in order to provide quality services with a maximum impact on public health outcomes. This book paves the way forward in terms of providing the first truly integrated educational resource for nurses. Such a significant contribution to the evolving speciality of integrated contraceptive and sexual healthcare will also enhance career pathways and opportunities for nurses. It also highlights the growing need for training and education programmes to be developed with the concept of integrated care in mind. Now is an opportune time to re-focus contraceptive and sexual health education programmes towards bringing the two specialities closer together.

Sarah and Alison's book will, therefore, be welcome, not only to nurses currently providing integrated models of contraceptive and sexual healthcare, but also to a much wider range of healthcare workers who provide care in either of the contraception or GUM specialities, as well as educationalists who will provide programmes of training to these practitioners.

Kevin Miles
Nurse Consultant & Hon Lecturer in Sexual Health
Camden Primary Care Trust/Centre for Sexual Health & HIV Research
University College London
April 2006

Preface

Sexual health and contraception services are becoming more integrated. It is more common these days to find contraceptive services being provided in hospital sexual health departments, and community contraception services are becoming increasingly involved in chlamydia and other STI (sexually transmitted infection) screening. In addition, with the new contract, many GP services are opting into providing basic sexual health screening as well as more specialist contraception services; and some pharmacists are providing emergency contraception and chlamydia screening. As health practitioners working in these fields it is useful to expand our knowledge across a wider range of areas. As a consequence we can provide a more holistic service for clients, destigmatise sexual and reproductive health, and reduce STI prevalence and unplanned pregnancy through improving access to these services.

This book aims to equip health practitioners with the knowledge they require to provide contraception and sexual health services, giving an overview of assessment for contraception and contraceptive methods, how to take a sexual health history, how to assess which swabs to take and how to take them, diagnosis and treatment regimes. It also gives an overview of other issues that can arise in this setting such as confidentiality issues, sexual assault and contact tracing.

Sarah Bekaert has a background in paediatrics and primary care; Alison White in gynaecology and sexual health. In their current roles as development nurses in City and Hackney Young People's Services they have developed pioneering community contraception and sexual health services, particularly with young people ('Choices E5, E9, N4 and N1'); projects have included a community young people's sexual health clinic offering testing, microscopy, diagnosis and treatment of most STIs, and contraceptive and counselling services; a joint sexual health and contraception clinic for young people with the local department of sexual health; and an emergency contraception drop-in clinic. We have written operational policy and patient group directions to support clinical work within nurse-led services. It has been a hard few years but very rewarding and we feel this book will be an essential reference for other clinicians embarking on, or already involved in, developing sexual health and contraception services.

Sarah Bekaert
Alison White
April 2006

Introduction

This book is a handbook for clinicians working at all levels in sexual and reproductive health. Combining both sexual health and contraceptive information, it combines both theoretical information and guidance on the practicalities of these specialities, e.g. swab-taking and the insertion and removal of certain contraceptive methods. As such it is an essential resource that can be referred to in day-to-day practice.

It covers the following areas:

Contraception:
- taking a contraceptive history and the rationale behind the assessment
- contraceptive methods, how they work, their indications, contraindications, side effects, drug interactions
- insertion and removal of contraceptive devices: subdermal, intrauterine, vaginal
- useful additional information for contraception provision such as a quick reference list of antibiotics and enzyme inducers that reduce the efficacy of the combined pill
- a guide to contraceptive methods that can be used when breastfeeding
- diagrams and charts: BMI (body mass index) chart, the menstrual cycle and diagrams of the male and female reproductive system.

Sexual health:
- taking a sexual health history
- an overview of STIs (sexually transmitted infections), their aetiology and prevalence
- diagnostic methods
- a comprehensive formulary for sexual health treatment drugs
- confidentiality issues
- contact tracing
- sexual assault.

The aim is for this book to bring all basic information required for a practitioner working in sexual and reproductive health together in a quick reference format.

The two sections within this book have been developed through the challenges and barriers we have faced as nurses while providing integrated services in a community setting. This book is meant as a guide only and should be adapted to each service area as applicable. It is also important to recognise in the areas of sexual and contraceptive health that rapid changes in the field mean that one will constantly have to keep updated.

What are integrated services?

The definition of sexual health in relation to providing a holistic framework includes the following services:

- contraception
- pregnancy
- abortion
- STIs
- sexual wellbeing
- HIV (human immunodeficiency virus).[1]

In recent times the term 'integrated services' has been used to describe various different levels of services and service provision. The term has been recognised in the Sexual Health Strategy 2001, which highlights the need to take a more holistic approach to sexual and reproductive healthcare.[2] Providing all sexual health services under one roof has been suggested as a model to ensure a more integrated approach to healthcare.[3]

Sexual health services need to be dealing with all aspects of sexual and reproductive health. It should be possible to access STI services via a family planning clinic and contraceptive services via a GU (genitourinary) clinic, whether provided on site or via integrated care pathways within a sexual health service network.[4]

This new way of looking at service provision has led to the review of non-mainstream service providers who have the potential to expand provision of sexual and reproductive health services. These services include general practitioners (GPs), pharmacists, abortion services, contraceptive services and other community-based stakeholders.

There are various interventions that these services have taken on, which include:

- chlamydia screening programme
- emergency contraception provision
- enhanced service provision
- condom distribution scheme.

As defined in the Sexual Health Strategy, models of service provision would be dependent on who is providing the service, their capacity and the skill mix within the team.

Overview of the Sexual Health and HIV Strategy

The Strategy[1] aims to:

- reduce the transmission of HIV and STIs
- reduce the prevalence of undiagnosed HIV and STIs
- reduce unintended pregnancy rates
- improve health and social care for people living with HIV
- reduce the stigma associated with HIV and STIs.

The Sexual Health and HIV Strategy divides sexual health provision into three main levels (*see* box); this can be used as a guide to the level of service you may be able to provide.

Definition of level of service provision

Level one
1 Sexual history and risk assessment.
2 Contraceptive information and services.
3 STI testing for women.
4 Assessment and referral of men with STI symptoms.
5 HIV testing and counselling.
6 Cervical cytology screening and referral.
7 Pregnancy testing and referral – hepatitis B immunisation.

Level two
1 Intrauterine device (IUD) insertion.
2 Contraceptive implant insertion.
3 Testing and treating STIs.
4 Partner notification.
5 Vasectomy.
6 Invasive STI.
7 Testing for men (until non-invasive tests are available).

Level three
Level three clinician teams will take responsibility for sexual health services needs assessment, for supporting provider quality, for clinical governance requirements at all levels and for providing specialist services. Services could include:

1 Outreach for STI prevention.
2 Outreach contraception services.
3 Specialised infections management, including co-ordination of partner notification.
4 Highly specialised contraception.
5 Specialised HIV treatment and care.

In addition Figure A shows the inter-relationships.

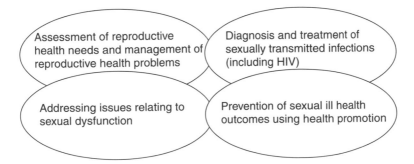

Figure A Inter-relationships of sexual health services.

Enhanced practice

It is encouraging that the public health White Paper *Choosing Health* sets out that sexual health services will increasingly be delivered by a flexible, multidisciplinary workforce, including nurses, youth workers, community workers and pharmacists.[5]

There has also been a review of the skill mix within teams, utilising the skills effectively so that there is ease of access, increased capacity, decreased waiting times and professional job satisfaction within services.

One of the disciplines that has advanced in this area of work is nursing. Nurses have been seen as a key tool in the implementation of and improvement in access to quality care services across the whole NHS. The rising profile of sexual and reproductive health nationally has led to the development of sexual and reproductive health nursing networks, developments and standardisation of nursing practice guidelines, and the development of nursing sexual health competency tools. There has also been a drive for increased provision of training for nurses who wish to take on an extended role within this field, examples being:

- the Royal College of Nursing (RCN) tools and training guide to provide a recognised qualification in Implanon and IUD fitting and removal
- supplementary and independent nurse prescribing courses.

Extending the role of the nurse and recognising its potential was highlighted as far back as 2000 in the government paper *The NHS Plan* and has led to developments of such roles as nurse specialists, nurse practitioners and nurse consultants.[6]

In addition there have been advancements in the use of healthcare support workers or assistants, recognising the need to formalise their roles and give them a professional footing within the field.[7]

Organisations such as the British Association for Sexual Health and HIV (BASHH) and the Faculty of Family Planning and Reproductive Health Care (FFPRHC) have recognised the advantages of integrating training opportunities and having nurse representatives within their systems. Nursing is being recognised as a competent profession in sexual and reproductive health. This means that nursing can now be held as an example of good practice in developing sexual health services and competencies in sexual and reproductive healthcare provision.

Links for sexual health competencies, sexual health patient group direction competency assessment from the National Prescribing Centre (NPC), and information on nurse prescribing can be found at the following websites:

- www.rcn.org.uk/members/downloads/contraceptionsexualhealth.pdf
- www.npc.co.uk/publications
- www.npc.co.uk/MeReC_Briefings/2003/briefing_no_23.pdf
- www.dh.gov.uk
- www.nmc-uk.org.

Associate nurse membership to BASHH and FFPRHC can be found at:

- www.bashh.org
- www.ffprhc.org.uk.

Snapshot of the City and Hackney model

City and Hackney Young People's Services (CHYPS) is a young person's sexual and reproductive health service for under 26 year olds. It is part of our Women and Young People's Services (WYPS).

Service provision includes:

- sex and relationship educational outreach
- contraceptive services with sexual health advice
- a comprehensive integrated sexual and reproductive health service providing under one roof:
  - microscopy
  - HIV testing
  - hepatitis testing and vaccination
  - counselling services
  - health adviser access (being trained in phlebotomy)
  - IUD and Implanon fitting and removal.

We work in a team where the nurses are dual trained and work autonomously, providing mostly nurse-led services, working to patient group directions or nurse prescribing. The doctors who support the services are from a dual-trained background; one is a GP with a special interest in sexual health. We also have development workers, administration staff and recently employed a healthcare support worker into the wider WYPS team.

We have therefore come from a place where integrated service provision has been mostly from a clinical base, providing as many services under one roof in a 'one-stop-shop' way of working but, where applicable, developing effective care pathways between interested organisations, agencies, departments and the local department of sexual health. This type of service provision is one example of a model of integrated service.

We were employed from teenage pregnancy strategy monies. Our remit was therefore to work towards reducing the incidence of unwanted and unplanned pregnancies in young people, according to the national strategy.

We were fortunate enough to have the support of the teenage pregnancy co-ordinators and the management team in recognising that our roles could be extended to being independent integrated service providers, using these extended roles to access hard-to-reach groups and to increase access to already existing services.

We therefore set about acquiring skills that would benefit the given population and allow for easier access into our service. Below is a list of processes that we went through in order to facilitate this.

- Reviewing job descriptions and working time and putting forward a proposal to increase the grades of the posts to accommodate for the extended roles. The RCN Sexual Health Competency Framework was used to underlie definitions of level of practice.
- Looking at areas outside of the clinical setting where our services could be utilised, e.g. youth clubs, colleges and in young people's hosted events.
- Having community bases from which to work in order to see clients *ad hoc* if the need arose, as well as working within clients' own environment when the skill would allow.

- Negotiating with stakeholders to provide services, for example emergency contraception provision or chlamydia urine testing.
- Discussing with pathology laboratories a possible increase in specimens to be sent to them and ensuring it was within the remit of the service level agreement.
- Liaising with the pharmacy department so as to inform them of situations in which drug administration and supply would be taking place.
- Holding departmental meetings with nurse manager and consultant leads to ensure that our practice would be supported.

In addition to the above we developed:

- appropriate sexual and reproductive health patient group directions to support our practice
- competency assessment tools for the use of sexual health patient group directions, adapted from the National Prescribing Centre framework
- operational guidelines and policy to support practice
- ease of communication with clients through mobile phones (for safety, client access to health education, advice and phone triage), which was publicised through service flyers and service publicity
- effective care pathways and referral pathways.

From an education viewpoint we undertook the following:

- Implanon fitting and removal training and practice
- IUD fitting training and practice
- bimanual examination training and practice
- nurse prescribing qualification
- Master's degree study relevant to practice
- being sources of referral and support for other practitioners and providing training and supervision to other health professionals.

These developments happened over a number of years and the aim was to become practitioners who were accessible and were able to provide a one-stop-shop service as far as our environment would allow. Our clients could phone us and ask for a service and we could arrange to meet them, preferably at a clinical location, in order to provide the service, or access them in their environment (e.g. college or youth setting). We also aimed to have recognised education and training that would enhance our practice and ensure that we were providing evidence-based care.

As practitioners we need to reflect on service needs, with whom you need to negotiate or inform in order to develop the service or your practice, and the skills and education needed to support any extended roles within the team.

The last word should be that whatever service provision is decided is that which is in the best interests of the client group you serve.

References

1 Department of Health (2001) *The National Strategy of Sexual Health and HIV*. HMSO, London.

2 Royal Society for the Promotion of Health (2004) *Choosing Health. A joint response from the Royal Society for the Promotion of Health.* Royal Society for the Promotion of Health, London.

3 French R (2005) *One-Stop Shop Versus Collaborative Integration: what is the best way of delivering sexual health services?* Unpublished.

4 Scottish Executive (2000) *Enhancing Sexual Wellbeing in Scotland: a sexual health and relationship strategy.* Scottish Executive.

5 FPA (2004) *Memorandum HA 08.* December. Health Select Committee, London.

6 DoH (2000) *The NHS Plan: a plan for investment, a plan for reform.* HMSO, London.

7 World Health Organization (2003) *Management of Sexually Transmitted Infections.* WHO, Geneva.

Section 1

Contraception

Chapter 1

Taking a contraceptive history

The aim of a good contraceptive history is to arrive at the best contraceptive method for the client, taking into consideration their medical, contraceptive and social history. This should be done in partnership with the client; the client is more likely to be successful in using a method if they have played an equal part in choosing it.

The client's history should be regularly reviewed and documented in the notes and an assessment made whether the client's current choice of contraception is still appropriate and safe.

Contraindications identified in this table will be explained in greater detail in the chapter relating to the specific method.

Increasingly a basic sexual health history is being included in a contraceptive history; how to take a sexual health history is covered in the sexual health section. The recommendation is that the health professional tailors the history-taking to best suit their area of practice.

A contraceptive history should include the points listed in the following table.

Menstrual history	Gives an idea of current patterns and possible existing conditions, e.g. fibroids with excessive bleeding, infection with postcoital or intermenstrual bleeding, polycystic ovarian syndrome (PCOS) with irregular bleeding.
	Once any pathology is identified and where possible treated, history may signpost to methods that can improve symptoms – e.g. the combined oral contraceptive pill (COC) to regulate bleeding, the intrauterine system (IUS) or injection (Depo-Provera) to ultimately improve bleeding – or ones to be avoided – e.g. intrauterine device (IUD) with already heavy periods.
When was the first day of the last period?	Amenorrhoea or irregular periods can indicate PCOS or pregnancy. Helps to identify when is the best time to start a method, i.e. 'quick-start' and seven days of extra precautions or wait for the next period (consider episodes of sexual intercourse and risk of pregnancy).
Are periods regular?	Irregular periods can indicate PCOS, anorexia, stress etc. If identifying when to fit an emergency coil, regular periods are required to accurately assess the safe time to insert the coil without possibly precipitating an abortion (up to five days after earliest ovulation).

How heavy is the bleeding?	Some women can have very heavy bleeding without realising it as they have nothing with which to compare. Very heavy bleeding can indicate the presence of fibroids; referral for a scan may be appropriate. Some hormonal contraceptive methods can improve heavy bleeding; indeed the Mirena IUS is licensed for menorrhagia as well as contraception.
How painful are periods?	Again some hormonal contraceptive methods can improve menstrual pain (dysmenorrhoea). Counselling may be appropriate as to which would be best; pain relief, e.g. a prostaglandin that relaxes smooth muscle (mefanemic acid), may be indicated.
	Client may mention other pain at other times in their cycle, which could be mittlesmirch, pathology (fibroids, cysts) or infection. The latter two should be eliminated through history-taking and appropriate investigations.
Premenstrual symptoms	Anovulatory methods can improve premenstrual symptoms.
When did periods start?	Early menarche has been associated with increased incidence of breast cancer.
Any gynaecological problems/operations	Will indicate which methods may be preferred or avoided, e.g. if only one uterine tube or history of ovarian cysts it is best to choose anovulatory method to reduce risk of ectopic pregnancy or further development of cysts.
Pregnancy history	Will elicit any pregnancy-induced problems such as hypertension and chloasma; the COC may induce these problems.
	Can lead to discussion re spacing children, avoiding pregnancy etc. with the longer-term contraceptive methods. If fitting an IUD a normal vaginal delivery will indicate the size of the cervical os. If there is a history of multiple caesarean section or previous ectopic pregnancy, increased likelihood of ectopic pregnancy.
Contraceptive history	Will give an idea of the methods already used and why discontinued; will give opportunity for counselling around these issues (discussing any misconceptions).
Cervical screening	Opportunity for health promotion and opportunistic screening.
Smoking	Opportunity for health promotion; nicotine is an enzyme inducer and smoking is a cofactor in the incidence of cervical neoplasia and cardiovascular disease.
Past medical history	Will indicate any contraindications or relative contraindications to certain contraceptive methods. For example:

Cardiovascular – COC use is associated with a small increased risk of venous thrombosis and is contraindicated in women who have a personal history of thrombosis.

Digestive – some digestive tract conditions can impede drug reabsorption, e.g. first-pass effect of COC and therefore contraceptive effect.

Epilepsy – some anti-epileptic drugs are enzyme inducers and reduce the efficacy of oral contraceptives.

Diabetes – increased risk of arterial disease, COC can be contraindicated.

Liver – consider the pharmacology of the drug and whether impaired liver function will affect drug availability.

Asthma – shock could precipitate an attack, e.g. injection, IUD insertion.

Cancer – with hormone-dependent cancers, hormonal contraceptive methods may exacerbate condition.

Headaches (specifically migraine)	Migraine is associated with a small increased risk of stroke; the COC is contraindicated in women who have migraine with focal aura.
Any STIs in the past	A client with a history of recurrent STIs and particularly pelvic inflammatory disease (PID) may have scarring in the uterine tubes; anovulatory methods may be preferred to avoid ectopic pregnancy. Use of condoms or Femidoms should be advocated.
Current illness	May contraindicate a method at present but could be reassessed in the future, e.g. COC is contraindicated if immobile due to increased risk of deep venous thrombosis (DVT).
Medication/herbal remedies	Will identify medications that can interfere with contraceptive action, e.g. enzyme inducers, some antibiotics. Herbal remedies can also interfere with the efficacy of contraception, e.g. St John's Wort is an enzyme inducer.
Allergies	Will indicate known allergies to constituents of contraceptive methods, e.g. copper in IUDs.
Family medical history	Primarily in first generation and then second: looking for predisposition to certain conditions that can present relative and possible absolute contraindications to certain contraceptive methods, e.g. cardiovascular disease, hypertension, diabetes, breast cancer.
Height/weight	An elevated body mass index (BMI) can be a contraindication to the COC. Low weight/anorexia can cause amenorrhoea/anovulatory cycles.

Blood pressure

An elevated blood pressure (BP) can be a contraindication to the COC as hypertension in COC users is the strongest risk factor for stroke.

Age

Under 16s need to be assessed for Fraser competency (*see* Chapter 8).

Age indicates fertility levels; reducing fertility levels can make less effective methods more reliable, e.g. diaphragm. Women over 35 who smoke should not be prescribed the COC due to increased arterial disease risk.

Chapter 2

Combined oral contraceptive methods

Combined oral contraceptive pill (COC)

Legal classification

Prescription-only medicine (POM).

Route of administration

Oral.

Efficacy

The combined oral contraceptive pill (COC) is 99% effective with careful use.

Formulations

Low strength

Loestrin 20 (Parke-Davis)
Norethisterone acetate 1 mg, ethinyloestradiol 20 micrograms (mcg)

Mercilon (Organon)
Desogestrel 150 mcg, ethinyloestradiol 20 mcg

Femodette (Schering)
Gestodene 75 mcg, ethinyloestradiol 20 mcg

Standard strength

Eugynon 30 (Schering)
Levonorgestrel 250 mcg, ethinyloestradiol 30 mcg

Logynon (Schering)
Six tablets: ethinyloestradiol 30 mcg, levenorgestrel 50 mcg
Five tablets: ethinyloestradiol 40 mcg, levenorgestrel 75 mcg
Ten tablets: ethinyloestradiol 30 mcg, levenorgestrel 125 mcg

Logynon ED (Schering)
As above plus seven inactive tablets

Microgynon 30 (Schering)
Levenorgestrel 150 mcg, ethinyloestradiol 30 mcg

Microgynon 30 ED (Schering)
As above plus seven inactive tablets

Ovranette (Wyeth)
Levenorgestrel 150 mcg, ethinyloestradiol 30 mcg

Trinordiol (Wyeth)
Six tablets: ethinyloestradiol 30 mcg, levenorgestrel 50 mcg
Five tablets: ethinyloestradiol 40 mcg, levenorgestrel 75 mcg
Ten tablets: ethinyloestradiol 30 mcg, levenorgestrel 125 mcg

Binovum (Janssen-Cilag)
Seven white tablets: ethinyloestradiol 35 mcg, norethisterone 500 mcg
Fourteen peach tablets: ethinyloestradiol 35 mcg, norethisterone 1 mg

Brevinor (Pharmacia)
Norethisterone 500 mcg, ethinyloestradiol 35 mcg

Loestrin 30 (Parke-Davis)
Norethisterone acetate 1.5 mg, ethinyloestradiol 30 mcg

Norimin (Pharmacia)
Norethisterone 1 mg, ethinyloestradiol 35 mcg

Ovysmen (Janssen-Cilag)
Norethisterone 500 mcg, ethinyloestradiol 35 mcg

Synphase (Pharmacia)
Seven blue tablets: ethinyloestradiol 35 mcg, norethisterone 500 mcg
Nine white tablets: ethinyloestradiol 35 mcg, norethisterone 1 mg
Five blue tablets: ethinyloestradiol 35 mcg, norethisterone 500 mcg

TriNovum (Janssen-Cilag)
Seven white tablets: ethinyloestradiol 35 mcg, norethisterone 500 mcg
Seven light peach tablets: ethinyloestradiol 35 mcg, norethisterone 750 mcg
Seven peach tablets: ethinyloestradiol 35 mcg, norethisterone 1 mg

Cilest (Janssen-Cilag)
Norgestimate 250 mcg, ethinyloestradiol 35 mcg

Marvelon (Organon)
Desogestrel 150 mcg, ethinyloestradiol 30 mcg

Yasmin (Schering)
Drospirenone 3 mg, ethinyloestradiol 30 mcg

Femodene (Schering)
Gestodene 75 mcg, ethinyloestradiol 30 mcg

Femodene ED (Schering)
As previous plus seven inactive tablets

Minulet (Wyeth)
Gestodene 75 mcg, ethinyloestradiol 30 mcg

Triadene (Schering)
Six beige tablets: ethinyloestradiol 30 mcg, gestodene 50 mcg
Five dark brown tablets: ethinyloestradiol 40 mcg, gestodene 70 mcg
Ten white tablets: ethinyloestradiol 30 mcg, gestodene 100 mcg

Triminulet (Wyeth)
Six beige tablets: ethinyloestradiol 30 mcg, gestodene 50 mcg
Five dark brown tablets: ethinyloestradiol 40 mcg, gestodene 70 mcg
Ten white tablets: ethinyloestradiol 30 mcg, gestodene 100 mcg

Norinyl-l (Pharmacia)
Norethisterone 1 mg, mestranol 50 mcg

How to take

With the COC pill one tablet is taken per day for 21 days followed by seven pill-free days. Ideally the pill should be taken at the same time every day, but if forgotten it should be taken within 12 hours of the normal time. If it goes beyond 12 hours the pill should still be taken, but it should be regarded as a missed pill and extra precautions should be used (see later for missed-pill rules) as well as taking the pill as normal. During the pill-free interval (PFI) the woman will have a short withdrawal bleed; even if the woman is still bleeding the next packet should be started after seven days.

Pharmacodynamics

The main actions of the COC are:

- prevents ovulation
- creates a cervical mucus plug
- impedes implantation.

Combined oral contraceptives containing a fixed amount of an oestrogen and a progestogen in each active tablet are termed monophasic. Those with varying amounts of the two hormones according to the stage of the cycle are termed biphasic and triphasic.

The oestrogen content ranges from 20 to 40 mcg and generally a preparation with the lowest oestrogen and progestogen content which gives good cycle control and minimal side effects in the individual is chosen.

All modern low-dose COCs contain ethinyloestradiol combined with a variety of progestogens. The latter are classified into two groups: levenorgestrel (LNG) and norethisterone (NET) (known as second-generation progestogens); and desogestrel (DSG), gestodene (GSD), drospirenone (DSP), cyproterone acetate (CPA), and norgestimate (NGM) (the second group allow more oestrogen dominance and are commonly known as third-generation progestogens).

The third-generation progestogens desogestrel, drospirenone and gestodene may be considered for women who experience progestogenic side effects (such as acne, headache, depression, weight gain, breast symptoms and break-through bleeding) as they, combined with ethinyloestradiol, are more oestrogen dominant. Women should be advised that desogestrel and gestodene may be associated with an increased risk of venous thromboembolism (VTE),[1-3] although there is recent evidence suggesting second-generation progestogens do not have these associated risks.[4,5]

Advantages

Advantages of the COC pill are:

- reliable and reversible
- reduced dysmenorrhoea and menorrhagia
- reduced incidence of premenstrual tension
- less symptomatic uterine fibroids and functional ovarian cysts
- less benign breast disease
- reduced risk of endometrial and ovarian cancer.

Absolute contraindications

- Pregnancy.
- Breastfeeding.
- Undiagnosed genital tract bleeding.
- Past or present circulatory disease.
- Liver disease.
- Cardiovascular and ischaemic heart disease.
- Lipid disorders.
- Oestrogen-dependent neoplasms.
- Migraine with aura.
- Cerebral haemorrhage.
- Transient ischaemic attacks.
- Obesity: BMI over 35 kg/m^2.*
- Severe diabetes mellitus with complications.
- Smokers over 35 years.
- Family history of arterial or venous disease in a first-degree relative aged less than 45 years.
- Acute episodes of Crohn's disease and ulcerative colitis.
- Allergy to pill constituent.
- History of serious condition affected by sex steroids or related to previous COC use.

Relative contraindications

- Sickle cell anaemia.
- Severe depression.
- Inflammatory bowel disease in remission.
- Diseases where HDL (high-density lipoprotein) is reduced, e.g. diabetes, hypertension.

- Splenectomy.
- Diseases whose drug treatment may affect the efficacy of the combined pill, e.g. epilepsy.
- Obesity: BMI 30–35 kg/m^2.*

Risk factors

Venous thromboembolism

The incidence of venous thromboembolism in healthy, non-pregnant women who are not taking an oral contraceptive is about 5 cases per 100 000 women per year. For those using combined oral contraceptives containing second-generation progestogens this incidence is about 15 per 100 000 women per year of use. Some studies have reported a greater risk of venous thromboembolism in women using preparations containing third-generation progestogens desogestrel and gestodene; the incidence in these women is about 25 per 100 000 women per year of use.[7]

Breast cancer

There is a slight increased risk of developing breast cancer while taking the COC and in the ten years after stopping (*see* table).

User status	Increased risk
Current user	24%
1–4 years after stopping	16%
5–9 years after stopping	7%
10-plus years an ex-user	No significant excess

Bear in mind that incidence of breast cancer increases with age and risk factors include early menarche and late age of first birth.[11]

Cervical cancer

The COC may act as a cofactor, speeding transition through all the stages of cervical intraepithelial neoplasia (CIN).[12]

---

* The World Health Organization Medical Eligibility Criteria (WHOMEC), taking research findings into consideration, recommends that the benefits of COC use by women with a BMI greater than 30 kg/m^2 outweigh the risks. No upper limit of BMI is given, but additional risk factors should be considered.[6] Hence, after counselling, women may still choose to use the COC pill. Guidance from the Faculty of Family Planning Clinical Effectiveness Unit states that, after counselling overweight women regarding the risks, they may choose the COC pill but should consider other methods.[7] The British National Formulary (BNF), on the other hand, states that a woman should not be given the COC if her BMI is greater than 39.[8] Guidelines by recognised experts in the field Professor Guillebaud[9] and Su Everett[10] state that with a BMI greater than 30 the COC pill should be used with caution, and if greater than 35 it is an absolute contraindication.

Migraine

Migraine with aura is a risk factor for ischaemic attack and is a contraindication to the COC.[13]

What exactly is an aura?
- Aura symptoms develop gradually before the headache, last up to one hour and resolve completely. Headache may be absent but the typical features of aura confirm the diagnosis.
- Most auras are visual, and often gradually spread across the visual field as a convex shape with a scintillating zigzag edge surrounding a bright scotoma. When asked to describe what they see, patients often draw a zigzag line in the air with a finger of either hand.
- Sensory symptoms may also occur; these are typically pins and needles spreading up one arm or affecting one side of the face, or aphasia.
- During the headache generalised blurred vision, spots in front of the eyes or photophobia are common and are not symptoms of an aura.[14]

Symptoms where the COC should be stopped

- Unusual, prolonged and severe headache.
- Aura.
- Speech disturbance.
- Numbness.
- Painful swelling in calf.
- Chest pain.
- Breathlessness.
- Severe abdominal pain.
- Immobilisation.
- Raised blood pressure.
- Detection of a significant new risk factor.

For how long can the COC be taken?

It is possible to continue taking the COC until age 51 (average age of menopause) as long as there are not any contraindications; beyond 51 years of age the related increased COC risks are usually unacceptable. With low fertility at this age, simple risk-free contraceptives are sufficient.

Drug interactions

Enzyme inducers

The effectiveness of COCs may be reduced by interaction with drugs that induce hepatic enzyme activity (the resultant reduced bioavailability leads to a reduced effect) (*see* box).

Well-known enzyme inducers

Carbamazepine
Griseofulvin
Modafinil
Nelfinavir
Nevirapine
Oxcarbazepine
Phenytoin
Phenobarbital
Primidone
Ritonavir
Topiramate
Rifabutin*
Rifampicin*
Barbiturates
Some antiretrovirals (*see* www.hiv-druginteractions.org for more information)
St John's Wort

*Rifampicin and rifabutin are such potent enzyme inducers that additional contraceptive precautions should be continued for at least four weeks after stopping.

For a short-term course of an enzyme-inducing drug, additional contraceptive precautions should be taken while taking the enzyme-inducing drug and for at least seven days after stopping it; if these seven days run beyond the end of a packet, the new packet should be started immediately without a break.

Antibiotics

Broad-spectrum antibiotics reduce gut flora and hinder contraceptive effect by interrupting reabsorption of metabolites from the gut (enterohepatic cycle) (*see* box).

Some common examples

Ampicillin, amoxicillin and related penicillins
Tetracyclines
Broad-spectrum cephalosporins

Additional contraceptive precautions should be taken while on a short course of broad-spectrum antibiotics and for seven days after stopping. If these seven days run beyond the end of a packet, the next packet should be started immediately without a break. If the antibiotic course exceeds three weeks, the bacterial flora develops antibiotic resistance and additional precautions are then unnecessary.

Side effects

Oestrogenic side effects

- Nausea.
- Dizziness.
- Cyclical weight gain.
- Vaginal discharge.
- Breast enlargement.
- Lost libido.

Progestogenic side effects

- Vaginal dryness.
- Sustained weight gain.
- Depression.
- Breast tenderness.

If clients have significant oestrogenic or progestogenic side effects, switch to an alternative COC in relation to the specific symptoms.

Starting routines

- On day 1 or 2 of period – no extra precautions required.
- Day 3 or later – seven days of extra precautions required (establish risk of pregnancy).
- Postpartum (not breastfeeding) – day 21 (low risk of thrombosis) – no extra precautions required.
- After termination of pregnancy (TOP) or miscarriage – same day or day 2, day 21 if beyond 24 weeks gestation – no extra precautions required.
- After higher-dose COC – instant switch or use condoms after PFI for seven days.
- After lower- or same-dose COC – after usual seven-day pill-free interval.
- After POP/contraceptive injection/implant – any day directly – no extra precautions required.
- After postcoital contraception – on day 2 of period (to be sure it is actual period).

Missed-pill rules

It has been felt that the World Health Organization (WHO) missed-pill recommendation for combined oral contraceptives, published in 2002, is too complex for many OC (oral contraceptive) users to understand. The recommendation included detailed and differing instructions depending on the number of pills missed and when they were missed. The 2004 WHO Expert Working Group simplified the missed-pill recommendation by giving one overarching instruction to women who miss any number of combined pills.[15] This guidance refers to combined OCs containing more than 20 mcg of the oestrogen ethinyloestradiol and one additional overarching instruction to women who miss three or more hormonal pills in a row:

- A woman who misses any number of hormonal pills should *take a hormonal pill as soon as possible and then continue taking one pill each day.* (If a woman follows a pill-taking schedule that involves starting on a certain day of the week, she must throw away the missed hormonal pills if she wants to maintain her schedule.)
- A woman who misses three or more hormonal pills in a row needs to take an additional step. She should *use condoms or abstain from sex until she has taken hormonal pills for seven days in a row.* A woman must take hormonal OCs for seven days continuously in order to prevent ovulation reliably.

It is particularly important to avoid extending the gap between taking hormonal pills. Therefore, if a woman misses three or more hormonal pills during the third week of the pill pack, she should finish only the hormonal pills in that pack and then start a new pack on the next day. Also, if a woman misses three or more hormonal pills in the first week of the pill pack and has had unprotected sex, the Expert Working Group advises that she may wish to consider using emergency contraception, because the risk of pregnancy in such a case could be substantial.

The 2004 Expert Working Group considered three to be the critical number of missed pills that should prompt women to take extra precautions. They based their judgement on evidence that up to nine days without hormones is not likely to lead to ovulation. Therefore, if a woman misses hormonal pills immediately before or after the seven-day hormone-free interval (that is, in either the third or first week of the pill pack), she could miss up to two hormonal pills – but not three – without risking pregnancy (two missed hormonal pills plus seven pill-free days equals nine days without hormones).

The more complex 2002 missed-pill recommendation instructed women to take extra precautions after missing two hormonal pills in a row, not three. Also, the 2002 recommendation for when to take extra precautions depended on when she missed the pills. For example, women who miss pills in the second or third week of the pill pack would have been taking hormonal pills for at least seven days previously, so they actually do not need to use additional contraception.

The 2004 guidance does not make such a distinction, however. The 2004 Expert Working Group's advice to use condoms or abstain from sex applies to all weeks of the pill pack. The Expert Working Group decided to sacrifice some scientific precision in the interest of simpler, easier to follow guidelines.

The guidance is more cautious for very-low-dose hormonal pills. Some COCs contain 20 mcg or less of the oestrogen ethinyloestradiol – a very low dose. If a woman misses any of these pills, WHO advises following the same rules as for other COCs, but with one key difference: a woman should take extra precautions after missing two hormonal pills, instead of after missing three.[15]

Biphasic and triphasic pills are not covered in detail here; they are not routinely prescribed in the UK as they do not have any significant advantage over monophasic pills. Regarding missed pills: due to varying quantities of hormones in each section, missing pills can prove complicated and it is best to encourage the client to seek professional advice immediately.

Diarrhoea and vomiting

Vomiting up to three hours after taking an oral contraceptive, or very severe diarrhoea, can interfere with its absorption. Additional precautions should therefore be used during and for seven days after recovery. If the vomiting or diarrhoea occurs during the last seven tablets the next pill-free interval should be omitted.

Breakthrough bleeding

Consider the following causes of breakthrough bleeding:

- disease – cervical and sexual health screening recommended
- disorders of pregnancy – retained products of conception
- missed pills
- medications/drugs
- severe diarrhoea and vomiting
- any cause that interferes with absorption in the gut.

Otherwise consider changing the COC to one with a different progestogen dose.

Yasmin (black triangle)

- The drospirenone in Yasmin acts as an anti-androgen and could be used to counter acne and PCOS. It also has diuretic properties.
- There are indications from clinical studies that Yasmin has a mild anti-mineralocorticoid effect.[16]
- Women using Yasmin and concomitant medications with the potential to increase serum potassium such as ACE (angiotensin-converting enzyme) inhibitors, angiotensin-II receptor antagonists, aldosterone antagonists, potassium-sparing diuretics or NSAIDs (non-steroidal anti-inflammatory drugs) used for long-term treatment should be tested for serum potassium during the first treatment cycle.

Dianette

(Each tablet contains 2 milligrams of the anti-androgen cyproterone acetate and 35 mcg of the oestrogen ethinyloestradiol.)

- Not licensed for contraception but acne and hirsuitism control. Women should be advised to switch to licensed oral contraceptive if continuing for contraceptive purposes once symptoms resolved.
- Dianette blocks androgen receptors. It also reduces androgen synthesis both by negative feedback effect on the hypothalamo-pituitary-ovarian systems and by the inhibition of androgen-synthesising enzymes.
- There is some epidemiological evidence that the incidence of VTE is higher in users of Dianette when compared to users of COCs with lower oestrogen content (<50 mcg).[17]

Tricycling

Tricycling is where three COC packets are taken consecutively followed by a seven-day PFI. This is suitable for women who wish to reduce withdrawal bleeds, high-conception-risk individuals, and during the use of enzyme-inducing drugs (consider also bicycling, four packets consecutively, shortening PFI).

Indications for tricycling:

- non-risk symptoms in PFI
- unacceptable/painful bleed in PFI
- maintenance treatment for endometriosis/epilepsy (may benefit from sustained levels of hormones)
- long-term enzyme-inducing therapy.

This is unlicensed usage.

Contraceptive patch

Legal classification

POM black triangle.

Route of administration

Transdermal.

Efficacy

The contraceptive patch is 99% effective.

Formulation

Each transdermal patch contains 6 mg norelgestromin (NGMN) and 600 mcg ethinyloestradiol.

How to take

Each patch is worn for seven days for three consecutive weeks followed by a patch-free week. It can be applied to the upper outer arm, upper torso (excluding breast), buttock or lower abdomen.

Pharmacodynamics/pharmacokinetics

The daily skin dose of 150 mg norelgestromin (the active metabolite of norgestimate) and 20 mg ethinyloestradiol produces blood levels similar to that from the combined pill Cilest but without diurnal fluctuation or the oral peak dose given to the liver.

The contraceptive patch works by:

- inhibiting ovulation
- altering cerivcal mucus so that it is impenetrable to sperm
- making the endometrium unfavourable to implantation.

Pharmacokinetic data suggest there is sufficient absorption of norelgestromin and ethinyloestrogen to maintain serum levels within the reference range for up to ten days.[18]

In one study into the efficacy of the contraceptive patch (1672 women, 72% completed the study) there were six pregnancies; four were in women weighing greater than 90 kg. Consequently the summary of product characteristics (SPC) suggests that the contraceptive patch is less effective in women weighing 90 kg or more.[19]

Advantages

- Client prefers combined method but is prone to forgetting pills.
- Reliable and reversible.
- Reduced dysmenorrhoea and menorrhagia.
- Reduced incidence of premenstrual tension.
- Less symptomatic fibroids and functional ovarian cysts.
- Less benign breast disease.
- Reduced risk of endometrial and ovarian cancer.

Absolute contraindications

- Pregnancy.
- Breastfeeding.
- Undiagnosed genital tract bleeding.
- Past or present circulatory disease.
- Liver disease.
- Cardiovascular and ischaemic heart disease.
- Lipid disorders.
- Oestrogen-dependent neoplasms.
- Migraine with aura.
- Cerebral haemorrhage.
- Transient ischaemic attacks.
- Obesity: BMI over 35 kg/m^2.
- Severe diabetes mellitus with complications.
- Smokers over 35 years.
- Family history of arterial or venous disease in a first-degree relative aged less than 45 years.
- Acute episodes of Crohn's disease and ulcerative colitis.
- Allergy to pill constituent.
- History of serious condition affected by sex steroids or related to previous COC use.

Relative contraindications

- Sickle cell anaemia.
- Severe depression.
- Inflammatory bowel disease in remission.
- Diseases where HDL is reduced.
- Splenectomy.
- Disease whose drug treatment affects the efficacy of the combined pill, e.g. tuberculosis (TB), epilepsy.
- Obesity: BMI 30–35 kg/m^2 or weight over 90 kg.

Drug interactions

Although first-pass metabolism in the liver is avoided with transdermal administration of hormones, the data on contraceptive efficacy with concurrent antibiotics are limited. The summary of product characteristics (SPC) advises use of barrier contraception when using antibiotics and for seven days after their discontinuation.

In the same way the SPC advises that during short-term enzyme inducer therapy and for 28 days afterwards additional contraception is still advised.[18]

Side effects

- Nausea.
- Breast tenderness and swelling.
- Headache.
- Local skin reaction.

Advice to clients

Absorption problems through diarrhoea and vomiting have no effect on this method's efficacy.

Starting routines

When there has been no hormonal contraceptive use in the preceding cycle

Contraception with the patch begins on the first day of menses. A single patch is applied and worn for one full week (seven days). The day the first patch is applied (day 1/start day) determines the subsequent change days. The patch change day will be on this day every week (cycle days 8, 15, 22 and day 1 of the next cycle). The fourth week is patch-free starting on day 22.

If cycle 1 starts after the first day of the menstrual cycle, a non-hormonal contraceptive should be used concurrently for the first seven consecutive days of the first treatment cycle only.

When switching from a combined oral contraceptive

Treatment with the hormonal patch should begin on the first day of withdrawal bleeding. If there is no withdrawal bleeding within five days of the last active (hormone-containing) tablet, pregnancy must be ruled out prior to the start of treatment. If therapy starts after the first day of withdrawal bleeding, a non-hormonal contraceptive must be used concurrently for seven days.

If more than nine days elapse after taking the last active oral contraceptive tablet, the woman may have ovulated and should, therefore, be advised to consult a physician before initiating treatment with the contraceptive patch. If intercourse has occurred during such an extended pill-free interval, the possibility of pregnancy risk should be considered.

When changing from a progestogen-only method

The woman may switch any day from the mini-pill/from an implant on the day of its removal/from an injectable when the next injection would be due, but a back-up barrier method of birth control must be used during the first seven days.

Following abortion or miscarriage

After an abortion or miscarriage that occurs before 20 weeks' gestation, the contraceptive patch may be started immediately. An additional method of contraception is not needed if the patch is started immediately. Be advised that ovulation may occur within ten days of an abortion or miscarriage.

After an abortion or miscarriage that occurs at or after 20 weeks' gestation, the patch may be started either on day 21 post-abortion or on the first day of the first spontaneous menstruation, whichever comes first. The incidence of ovulation on day 21 post-abortion (at 20 weeks' gestation) is not known.

Following delivery

Users who choose not to breastfeed can start contraceptive therapy with the patch no sooner than four weeks after childbirth. When starting later, the woman should be advised to use a barrier method in addition to the patch for the first seven days. However, if intercourse has already occurred, pregnancy should be excluded before the actual start of the patch or the woman has to wait for her first menstrual period.[19]

Missed-patch rules

- If a patch detaches for less than one day (up to 24 hours) then it should be replaced with a new patch immediately; additional contraception is unnecessary. The next patch should be changed on the usual change day.
- If the patch has been detached for 24 hours or more then a new patch should be applied and a new cycle commenced; additional contraception is required for seven days.
- If patch change days are delayed at the start of the patch cycle, a new patch should be applied immediately; additional contraception should be used for seven days (if there is a prolonged delay in the change of patch, emergency contraception may be required).

- If the patch is delayed in the middle of a cycle for up to 48 hours the client should apply a new patch immediately. The next patch should be applied on the usual change day; if the patch has been worn correctly for the preceding seven days then no additional contraception is required.
- If the patch is delayed for more than 48 hours mid-cycle the client should commence a new patch immediately; there will be a new change day and additional contraception needed for seven days.

References

1 Spitzer WO, Lewis MA, Heinemann LAJ, Thorogood M and MacRae KD (1996) Third generation oral contraceptives and risk of venous thromboembolitic disorders: an international case control study. *BMJ.* **312**: 83–8.

2 Jick H, Jick SS, Gurewich V, Myers MW and Vasilakis C (1995) Risk of idiopathic cardiovascular death among non fatal venous thromboembolism in women using oral contraceptive with differing progestogen components. *Lancet.* **346**: 1589–93.

3 Farley TMM, Meirik O, Chang I *et al.* (1995) World Health Organization collaborative study of cardiovascular disease and steroid hormone contraception. Effect of different progestogens in low oestrogen oral contraceptives on venous thromboembolic disease. *Lancet.* **346**: 1582–8.

4 Farmer RDT, Laurenson RA, Thompson CR, Kennedy JG and Hambleton IR (1997) Population based study of risk of venous thromboembolism associated with various oral contraceptives. *Lancet.* **349**: 83–8.

5 Lawreson R and Farmer R (2000) Venous thromboembolism and combined oral contraceptives: does the type of progestogen make a difference? *Contraception.* **62**(2): 21–8.

6 World Health Organization (WHO) (2000) *Medical Eligibility Criteria for Contraceptive Use.* WHO, Geneva.

7 Royal College of Obstetricians and Gynaecologists (RCOG) (2004) *Venous Thromboembolism and Hormonal Contraception Guidance (RCOG Clinical Green Top Guidance).* RCOG, London.

8 British National Formulary (BNF) (2004). **47**. March. www.BNF.org

9 Guillebaud J (2003) *Contraception: your questions answered.* Churchill Livingstone, London.

10 Everett S (2004) *Handbook of Contraception and Family Planning.* Ballière Tindall, Edinburgh.

11 Collaborative Group on Hormonal Factors in Breast Cancer (2002) Breast cancer and breastfeeding: collaborative reanalysis of individual data from 47 epidemiological studies in 30 countries, including 50,302 women with breast cancer and 96,973 women without the disease. *Lancet.* **360**: 187–95.

12 Ursin G, Peters RK, Henderson BE *et al.* (1994) Oral contraceptive use and adenocarcinoma of cervix. *Lancet.* **344**: 1390–4.

13 MacGregor EA (2001) *Hormonal Contraception and Migraine.* Faculty of Family Planning and Reproductive Health Care Factsheet. Royal College of Obstetricians and Gynaecologists, London.

14 Guillebaud J (2004) *Contraception Today.* Martin Dunitz, London.

15 WHO Expert Working Group (2004) *Selected Practice Recommendations for Contraceptive Use.* WHO, Geneva.

16 Electronic Medicines Compendium (2005) Yasmin film-coated tablets. www.emc.medicines.org.uk

17 Electronic Medicines Compendium (2004) Dianette. www.emc.medicines.org.uk

18 Electronic Medicines Compendium (2003) Evra transdermal patch. www.emc.medicines.org.uk

19 Faculty of Family Planning and Reproductive Health Care Clinical Effectiveness Unit (2004) New product review September 2003: Norelgestromin/ethinyl oestradiol transdermal contraceptive system (Evra). *Journal of Family Planning and Reproductive Health Care.* **30**(1): 43–5.

Chapter 3

Progestogen-only methods

Progestogen-only pill (POP)

Legal classification

POM.

Route of administration

Oral.

Efficacy

The progestogen-only pill (POP) is between 96% and 99% effective.

Formulations

Cerazette (Organon)
Tablets: desogestrel 75 mcg

Femulen (Pharmacia)
Tablets: etynodiol diacetate 500 mcg

Micronor (Jannsen-Cilag)
Tablets: norethisterone 350 mcg

Microval (Wyeth)
Tablets: levenorgestrel 30 mcg

Neogest (Schering Health)
Tablets: norgestrel 75 mcg

Norgeston (Schering Health)
Tablets: levenorgestrel 30 mcg

Noriday (Pharmacia)
Tablets: norethisterone 350 mcg

How to take

One tablet a day, at the same time each day.

Pharmacodynamics

The POP discourages implantation of a fertilised ovum by altering the endometrium. Cervical mucus viscosity is also changed which may render the passage of sperm less likely. In some cases it also prevents ovulation (in at least 60% of cycles).[1] The POP is absorbed from the gastrointestinal tract and metabolised in the liver.

Indications

- Where COC contraindicated:
  - smokers over 35 years
  - hypertension
  - migraine
  - diabetes
  - sickle cell anaemia
  - obesity (indication for Cerazette).
- Breastfeeding.
- Preferred method.

Contraindications

- Sex-steroid-dependent cancers.
- Past ectopic pregnancy (indication for Cerazette: a predominantly anovulatory POP).
- Malabsorption syndromes.
- Functional ovarian cysts.
- Active liver disease.
- Severe arterial disease.
- Porphyria.
- If using enzyme inducers.

Drug interactions

Reduced efficacy and increased incidence of breakthrough bleeding have been associated with concomitant use of oral contraceptives and rifampicin. A similar association has been suggested with oral contraceptives and barbiturates, phenytoin sodium, ampicillin, tetracyclines and griseofulvin.

The herbal remedy St John's Wort *(Hypericum perforatum)* should not be taken concomitantly with the POP as this could potentially lead to a loss of contraceptive effect; it is common practice to recommend two POPs per day for women taking enzyme inducers.[2]

Side effects

Side effects are usually self-limiting and of relatively short duration.

- Nausea.
- Vomiting.
- Headache.
- Dizziness.
- Breast discomfort/breast changes.
- Depression.
- Skin disorders.
- Disturbance of appetite.
- Weight changes.
- Changes in libido.
- Chloasma.
- Rash.
- Depression.
- Menstrual irregularities.

It is important that patients are advised that while using the POP they may experience variation in cycle length and that they should continue taking a tablet every day whether they have a period or not.

Starting routines

Day 1 or 2 of period

No extra precautions required.

The POP can be started mid-cycle as long as pregnancy risk has been excluded; however, the client should be advised that it will not provide contraception until it has been taken for seven consecutive days and extra precautions should be used up until that time.

Changing from another hormonal contraceptive

Start the POP on the day following completion of the previous contraceptive; for the COC pill omit the pill-free interval (or in the case of the ED (everyday) pill, omitting the inactive pills). No extra contraceptive precautions are required.

Postpartum administration

The POP can be started on the 21st day after childbirth. This will ensure the patient is protected immediately. If there is any delay in taking the first dose, contraception may not be established until seven days after the first tablet has been taken. In these circumstances, patients should be advised that barrier contraceptive precautions are necessary.

After miscarriage or abortion

Patients can take the POP on the day after miscarriage or abortion, in which case no additional contraceptive precautions are required.

Missed tablets

If a tablet is missed within three hours of the correct dosage time, then the missed tablet should be taken as soon as possible; this will ensure that contraceptive protection is maintained. If one (for longer than three hours) or more tablets are missed, it is recommended that the patient takes the last missed tablet as soon as possible and continues to take the rest of the tablets as usual. Additional means of contraception (non-hormonal) should be used for the next two days.[3]

Diarrhoea and vomiting

Additional contraceptive measures (non-hormonal) should be employed during the period of gastrointestinal upset and for the next seven days.

Weight

It has become accepted practice for women over 70 kg to take two POPs a day; this is based on studies that suggested that the failure rate of POPs was higher with increasing weight. It may be better to give the anovulatory Cerazette to these clients.

Cerazette

Cerazette contains 75 mg desogestrel and stops ovulation in 97% of cycles.[4] It can be used where a COC is contraindicated but a pill method with greater efficacy than an ordinary POP is desired, e.g. a woman over 70 kg, a history of ectopic pregnancy or ovarian cysts. It has a 12-hour window period.

Parenteral progestogen-only contraception

Legal classification

POM.

Route of administration

Parenteral.

Efficacy

The efficacy of parenteral progestogen-only contraception is 99–100%.

Formulation

Depo-Provera (Pharmacia)
Medroxyprogesterone acetate 150 mg/ml prefilled syringe (the only injectable currently licensed by the Committee on Safety of Medicines for long-term use).

How to take

Doses should be given once every 12 weeks by deep intramuscular (IM) injection. Care should be taken to ensure that the depot injection is given into the muscle tissue, preferably the gluteus maximus, but other muscle tissue such as the deltoid may be used.

Pharmacodynamics

Each millilitre of suspension contains 150 mg medroxyprogesterone acetate.

Medroxyprogesterone acetate is a long-acting progestational steroid and exerts anti-oestrogenic, anti-androgenic and antigonadotrophic effects. The long duration of action results from its slow absorption from the injection site. The plasma half-life is about six weeks after a single intramuscular injection.

Indications

- Women preferring highly effective non-oral method.
- Women with heavy and/or prolonged bleeding.
- Women with unacceptable premenstrual symptoms.
- Preferred method.

Absolute contraindications

- Past or current severe arterial disease (links between low oestrogen and lowered HDL cholesterol).
- Severe risk factors for osteoporosis.
- Recent breast cancer.
- Recent trophoblastic disease.
- Acute porphyria.

Relative contraindications

- Arterial risk.
- Active liver disease.
- Non-acute porphyria.
- Sex-steroid-dependent cancer in complete remission.

Drug interactions

- Aminoglutethimide administered concurrently with Depo-Provera may significantly depress the bioavailability of Depo-Provera.
- Enzyme inducers: the clearance of medroxyprogesterone acetate is approximately equal to the rate of hepatic blood flow, therefore it is unlikely that drugs which induce hepatic enzymes will significantly affect the kinetics of medroxyprogesterone acetate. Therefore, no dose adjustment is recommended in patients receiving drugs known to affect hepatic metabolising enzymes.[1]

Side effects

- Menstrual irregularities.
- Delayed return of fertility.
- Weight gain.
- Headaches.
- Feeling bloated.
- Depression.
- Mood swings.

Menstrual irregularity

The administration of Depo-Provera usually causes disruption of the normal menstrual cycle. Bleeding patterns include amenorrhoea, irregular bleeding and spotting, and prolonged episodes of bleeding. If abnormal bleeding persists or is severe, appropriate investigation should take place to rule out the possibility of organic pathology; excessive or prolonged bleeding can be controlled by the co-administration of oestrogen. This may be delivered in the form of a low-dose (30 mcg oestrogen) combined oral contraceptive. Oestrogen therapy may need to be repeated for one to two cycles. Long-term co-administration of oestrogen is not recommended.[5]

If unacceptable bleeding occurs towards the end of the three months the next injection could be given earlier, but not less than four weeks since the last dose.[3]

Return of fertility

Pregnancies have occurred as early as 14 weeks after a preceding injection; however, in clinical trials, the mean time to return of ovulation was 5.3 months following the preceding injection. Eighty-three per cent of women may be expected to conceive within 12 months of the first 'missed' injection; the median time to conception is 10 months after the last injection.[1]

Weight gain

There is a tendency for women to gain weight while on Depo-Provera therapy. Studies indicate that over the first one to two years of use, average weight gain was 5–8 lb. Women completing four to six years of therapy gained an average of 14–16.5 lb. There is evidence that weight is gained as a result of increased fat and is not secondary to an anabolic effect or fluid retention.[1]

Starting routines

First injection

To provide contraceptive cover in the first cycle of use, an injection of 150 mg IM should be given during the first five days of a normal menstrual cycle. If the injection is carried out according to these instructions, no additional contraceptive cover is required. If given later after establishing whether there is a pregnancy risk, seven days of extra precautions are required.

Following COC/patch, POP or sub-dermal method

Immediate follow-on with no added precautions; no pill-free interval for COC.

Postpartum

If not breastfeeding or after second-trimester abortion: day 21.

If the puerperal woman is breastfeeding, the initial injection should be given no sooner than six weeks postpartum, when the infant's enzyme system is more fully developed.

There is evidence that women prescribed Depo-Provera in the immediate puerperium can experience prolonged and heavy bleeding. Because of this, the drug should be used with caution in the puerperium.

After miscarriage or first-trimester abortion

By day 7 or later if no pregnancy risk plus seven days extra precautions.

Overdue injections

The World Health Organization advises that a 'late' Depo-Provera injection can be given up to 14 weeks.[6] However, as there have been reported conceptions as early as the end of the 13th week, the following is recommended by contraceptive expert practitioners.

- From day 85 to 91 (13th week): injection plus condoms for next seven days.
- From day 92 to 98 (14th week): injection plus emergency contraception as necessary plus extra precautions for seven days.
- Beyond day 98: next injection delayed until 14 days of safe contraception or abstinence, negative pregnancy test and seven days of extra precautions.[3]

Loss of bone mineral density

Loss of bone mineral density (BMD) may occur in females of all ages who use Depo-Provera injection long term. Depo-Provera reduces serum oestrogen levels and is associated with loss of BMD due to the known effect of oestrogen deficiency on the bone remodelling system. Bone loss is greater with increasing duration of use and appears to be at least partially reversible after Depo-Provera injection is discontinued and ovarian oestrogen production increases. Therefore a risk/benefit assessment, which also takes into consideration other causes of BMD loss, should be considered, e.g. family history of osteoporosis, smoking, breastfeeding.

Adolescence is a critical period of bone accretion; it is unknown if use of Depo-Provera injection by adolescent women will reduce peak bone mass and increase the risk for osteoporotic fracture in later life. Current best practice is that for adolescents, Depo-Provera may be used, but only after other methods of contraception have been discussed with the patients and considered to be unsuitable or unacceptable.[7]

In women of all ages, careful re-evaluation of the risks and benefits of treatment should be carried out in those who wish to continue use for more than two years. In women with significant lifestyle and/or medical risk factors for osteoporosis, other methods of contraception should be considered prior to use of Depo-Provera.

Implant

Legal classification

POM.

Route of administration

Subdermal.

Efficacy

The implant is over 99% effective.

Formulation

Implanon (Organon)
Subdermal implant containing 68 mg etonogestrel, dispersed in a matrix and covered by a rate-limiting membrane. Implanon lasts three years.

How to take

Implanon should be inserted (and removed) by a trained professional. A single 40 mm rod, 2 mm in diameter, it is inserted subdermally straight from a dedicated sterile preloaded applicator via a wide-bore needle.

See diagram of insertion and removal technique as recommended by the manufacturer, Organon (Figure 3.1a–r, reproduced courtesy of Organon).

How to insert Implanon

- Insertion of Implanon should be performed under aseptic conditions, and only by a clinician who is familiar with the procedure.
- Insertion of Implanon is performed with the specially designed applicator. The use of this applicator differs substantially from that of a classical syringe. A drawing of a dismantled applicator and its individual components (e.g. cannula, obturator and needle with double-angled bevel) is shown in Figure 3.1r to clarify their specific functions.
- The procedure used for insertion of Implanon is opposite to giving an injection. When inserting Implanon the obturator must remain fixed while the cannula (needle) is retracted from the arm. For normal injections the plunger is pushed and the body of the syringe remains fixed.

- Allow the subject to lie on her back with her non-dominant arm (the arm which the woman does not use for writing) turned outwards and bent at the elbow.
- Implanon should be inserted at the inner side of the upper arm (non-dominant arm) about 6–8 cm above the elbow crease in the groove between the biceps and the triceps (sulcus bicipitalis medialis).
- Mark the insertion site.
- Clearn the insertion site with a disinfectant.
- Anaesthetise with an anaesthetic spray, or with 2 ml of lidocaine (1%) applied just under the skin along the 'insertion canal'.
- Remove the sterile disposable applicator carrying Implanon from its blister and remove the needle shield.
- Always hold the applicator in the upward position (i.e. with the needle pointed upwards) until the time of insertion. This is to prevent the implant from dropping out.
- Visually verify the presence of the implant inside the metal part of the cannula (the needle). The implant can be seen as a white tip inside the needle. If the implant protrudes from the needle, return it to its original position by tapping against the plastic part of the cannula. Keep the needle and the implant sterile. If contamination occurs, a new package with a new sterile applicator must be used.
- Stretch the skin around the insertion site with thumb and index finger (Figure 3.1a).
- Insert only the tip of the needle, slightly angled (~20°) (Figure 3.1b).

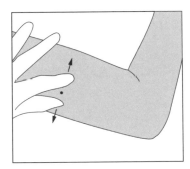

Figure 3.1a

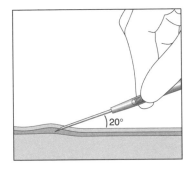

Figure 3.1b

- Release the skin.
- Lower the applicator to a horizontal position (Figure 3.1c).
- Lift the skin with the tip of the needle, but keep the needle in the subdermal connective tissue (Figure 3.1d).
- Gently insert, while lifting the skin, the needle to its full length without using force.
- Keep the applicator parallel to the surface of the skin.
- When the implant is placed too deeply the removal can be hampered later on.
- Break the seal of the applicator (Figure 3.1e).
- Turn the obturator 90° (Figure 3.1f).

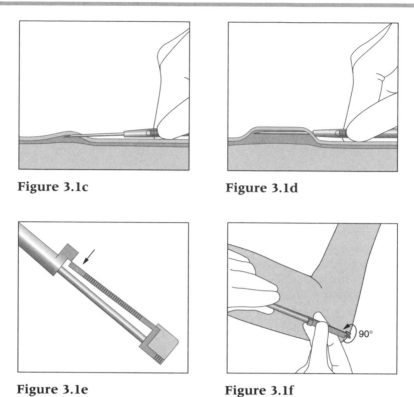

Figure 3.1c   Figure 3.1d

Figure 3.1e   Figure 3.1f

- Fix the obturator with one hand against the arm and with the other hand slowly retract the cannula (needle) out of the arm (Figure 3.1g).
- Never push against the obturator.
- Check the needle for the absence of the implant. After retraction of the cannula, the grooved tip of the obturator should be visible (Figure 3.1h).

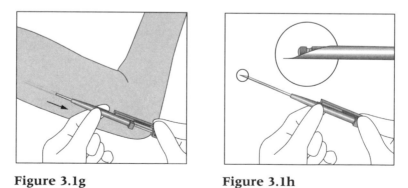

Figure 3.1g   Figure 3.1h

How to remove Implanon

- Removal of Implanon should only be performed by a clinician who is familiar with the removal technique.

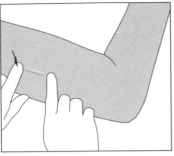

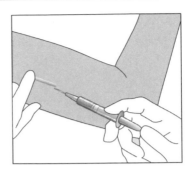

Figure 3.1i   **Figure 3.1j**

- Locate the implant by palpation and mark the distal end. In case that Implanon can not be palpated it is strongly advised to locate the implant by either ultrasound (USS) or magnetic resonance imaging (MRI). Prior to the application of USS and MRI for the localisation of Implanon it is recommended to consult Organon for the proper instructions (Figure 3.1i).
- A non-palpable implant should always first be localised by USS (or MRI) and subsequently be removed under the guidance of USS.
- Wash the area and apply a disinfectant.
- Anaesthetise the arm with 0.5–1 ml lidocaine (1%) at the site of incision, which is just below the distal end of the implant. Note: Apply the anaesthetic under the implant. Application above the implant makes the skin swell, which may cause difficulties in locating the implant (Figure 3.1j).
- Make an incision of 2 mm in length in the longitudinal direction of the arm at the distal end of the implant (Figure 3.1k).
- Gently push the implant towards the incision until the tip is visible. Grasp the implant with forceps (preferably 'mosquito' forceps) and remove it (Figure 3.1l).

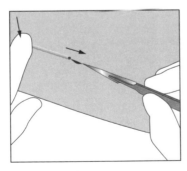

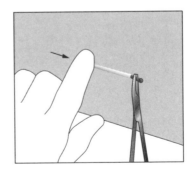

Figure 3.1k   **Figure 3.1l**

- If the implant is encapsulated, an incision into the tissue sheath should be made and the implant then removed with forceps (Figures 3.1m, n).
- If the tip of the implant is not visible, gently insert a forceps into the incision and grasp the implant (Figures 3.1o, p). With a second forceps carefully dissect the tissue around the implant. The implant can then be removed (Figure 3.1q).
- Close the incision with a butterfly closure.

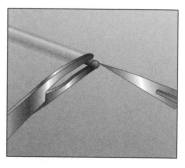

Figure 3.1m

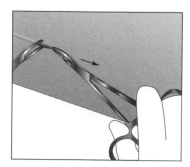

Figure 3.1n

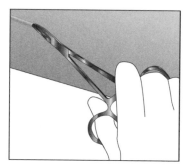

Figure 3.1o

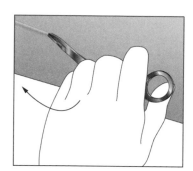

Figure 3.1p

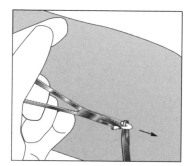

Figure 3.1q

- Apply sterile gauze with a pressure bandage to prevent bruising.
- There have been occasional reports of displacement of the implant; usually this involves minor movement relative to the original position. This may somewhat complicate removal.

Pharmacodynamics

Implanon exerts its contraceptive effect by progestogenic means:

- ovulation inhibition
- mucus formation at the cervix
- altering the endometrium to make it non-receptive to implantation.

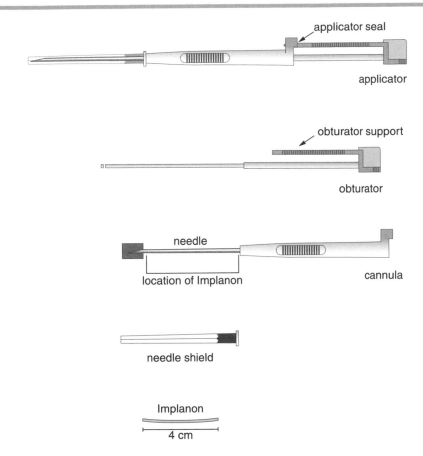

applicator seal

applicator

obturator support

obturator

needle

location of Implanon

cannula

needle shield

Implanon

4 cm

Figure 3.1r

Within one day after injection the serum blood concentrations of etonogestrel are achieved to inhibit ovulation (90 pg/ml). Maximum concentrations of this hormone are reached after four days, but these are 20% of the concentration achieved with a COC pill containing 150 mg desogestrel. Etonogestrel appears to inhibit luteinising hormone without affecting FSH (follicle-stimulating hormone) production, with the result that preovulatory follicles continue to produce oestradiol; therefore there are no concerns that this method may predispose to a reduced bone mineral density or cardiovascular disease.[8]

Enzyme inducers

If enzyme inducer drug treatment is necessary, additional contraceptive precautions are recommended. One option is to prescribe an added daily Cerazette tablet (unlicensed use).[3]

Indications

- Long acting.
- Highly effective.
- Reversible (more than 90% of women ovulate within 30 days after removal).

- Requires little user compliance.
- Independent of intercourse.
- Oestrogen free.
- Anovulant.

Absolute contraindications

- Any adverse effect of COC not related to oestrogen component, e.g. progestogen allergy, liver adenoma.
- Recent breast cancer not yet clearly in remission.
- Acute porphyria.
- Recent trophoblastic disease until hCG (human chorionic gonadotrophin) is undetectable in blood as well as urine.
- Pregnancy.
- Undiagnosed genital tract bleeding.
- Hypersensitivity to any component.

Relative contraindications

- Latent acute porphyria.
- Sex-steroid-dependent cancer in complete remission for two years.
- Enzyme inducers (Cerazette can be used in addition).
- Past symptomatic functional ovarian cysts (may recur).
- Risk factors for arterial disease.
- Current liver disorder.
- Chronic severe systemic diseases.

Side effects

- Irregular bleeding.*
- Abdominal pain.*
- Acne.
- Headache.
- Breast pain.
- Dizziness.
- Mood changes.
- Libido decrease.
- Hair loss.
- May induce mild insulin resistance.

Weight

In studies serum levels of etonogestrel were lower in heavier women using the implant, but there were no failures whatever the BMI. Serum steroid

---

* Overall contraceptive implant users appear to experience less bleeding than non-users and may have an improvement in reported dysmenorrhoea. One study suggested that 84% of women suffering from dysmenorrhoea prior to use of an implant noticed complete resolution of this problem.[8] Implanon users appear to experience less bleeding but have a more variable pattern.

concentrations with Implanon appear to be greater than the minimum dose required to inhibit ovulation, even in women with a high BMI. Current best practice is to replace the implant at two years in young fertile women weighing over 100 kg if they start cycling regularly in the third year.[3]

Starting routines

No previous hormonal contraception

Inserted during first five days of cycle.

Parturition or abortion in second trimester

Start 21–28 days after delivery or abortion.

Abortion in first trimester

Inserted immediately.

No sexual intercourse since period or following POP

At any time plus seven days of extra precautions.

Using COC, Cerazette or contraceptive injection

Can be inserted any time with no extra precautions.

Breastfeeding

Insert after six weeks.

NB: For nurses wishing to train to fit and remove Implanon you need to have a family planning qualification, undergo theoretical training (your local Organon representative will help you organise this) and have local practical training with a Faculty of Family Planning teaching doctor. The RCN produces a training guide with a proforma to complete; once this is achieved the RCN will issue a certificate of competence.

Progestogen-only emergency contraception (POEC)

Legal classification

POM.

Route of administration

Oral.

Efficacy

Up to 95% of pregnancies are prevented.

Formulation

Levonelle 1500 (Schering Health)
Levenorgestrel (LNG) 1500 mcg.
Can be sold to women over 16 years as 'Levonelle' (P).

How to take

Effective if taken within 72 hours of unprotected intercourse; taking the dose as soon as possible increases efficacy. May be used between 72 and 120 hours after unprotected intercourse (unlicensed use) but efficacy decreases with time.

Randomised controlled trials confirm the effectiveness of two 750 mg LNG tablets taken 12 hours apart, within 72 hours of unprotected sexual intercourse (UPSI). The pharmacokinetics of LNG are the same when the second dose is taken 12 or 24 hours after the first and the summary of product characteristics suggests the two doses can be given 12–16 hours apart.[9]

However, serum levels of LNG are similar following a single 1.5 mg dose and following the conventional regime of two 0.75 mg doses taken 12 hours apart. A trial by the World Health Organization compared single and divided doses of LNG taken within 120 hours of UPSI; no differences in pregnancy rates between these regimens were identified.[10] Results from a recent clinical study showed that two 750 mcg LNG tablets taken at the same time (and within 72 hours of unprotected sex) prevented 84% of expected pregnancies (compared with 79% when the tablets were taken 12 hours apart).[1]

Current recognised practice is to advise both tablets be taken together, and Levonelle 1500 (one tablet containing 1500 mcg LNG) is being phased in.

Levonelle is unlicensed for use more than once in a menstrual cycle. Failure rates of 0.8% per treatment cycle have been identified when Levonelle has been used more than once. Nevertheless Levonelle can be used more than once in a cycle if clinically indicated.[9]

Pharmacodynamics

The precise mode of action of Levonelle is not known; however, it is thought to work mainly by preventing ovulation and fertilisation if intercourse has taken place in the preovulatory phase, when the likelihood of fertilisation is at its highest. It may also cause endometrial changes that discourage implantation. Levonelle is not effective once the process of implantation has begun.[1]

Indications

- Unprotected sexual intercourse.
- Potential contraceptive failure.

Contraindications

There are very few absolute contraindications to Levonelle.

- Pregnancy (although the progestogen will not harm the foetus).
- Proven severe acute allergy to a constituent.
- Active acute porphyria with past attack.
- Active severe liver disease.

Drug interactions

Enzyme inducers

Current advice is that two tablets (1.5 mg LNG) are followed 12 hours later by a single tablet (0.75 mg LNG); this is outside the product licence.

Warfarin

Caution is advised when prescribing Levonelle for women using warfarin. It has been observed that the anticoagulant effects of warfarin can be decreased or increased following use.[9]

Side effects

- If vomiting occurs within three hours of taking Levonelle a replacement dose can be given.
- Levonelle failure is not thought to increase the risk of foetal abnormality.

Treatment failure rate

The treatment failure rate is the percentage of women who get pregnant despite using Levonelle. Reported failure rates of Levonelle range from 1% to 3%. As the overall risk of pregnancy following one act of UPSI at any time in the menstrual cycle is only 2–4%, the vast majority of women will not become pregnant following UPSI, even without using Levonelle. For this reason the efficacy of Levonelle may be more usefully expressed as the proportion of expected pregnancies prevented. Used within 72 hours of UPSI, Levonelle will prevent up to 86% of expected pregnancies (*see* table).[3,9]

Coitus to treatment interval	% of expected pregnancies prevented
Less than 24 hours	95
25–48 hours	85
49–72 hours	58
72–120 hours	Not calculated (small numbers)

Advanced provision of POEC

Advanced provision of POEC can be offered to appropriate cases with instructions on use and how to access services if side effects occur; however, this is unlicensed usage.

References

1 Electronic Medicines Compendium (2005) www.emc.medicines.org.uk
2 Faculty of Family Planning and Reproductive Health Care Clinical Effectiveness Unit (2004) Contraceptive choices for breastfeeding women. *Journal of Family Planning and Reproductive Health Care.* **30**(3): 181–9.
3 Guillebaud J (2004) *Contraception Today* (5e). Martin Dunitz, London.
4 Faculty of Family Planning and Reproductive Health Care (FFPRHC) (2003) *New Product Review. Desogestrel Only Pill (Cerazette).* April. FFPRHC, London.
5 Porter C (2002) Bleeding patterns and progestogen only contraception. *Journal of Family Planning and Reproductive Health Care.* **28**(4): 178–81.
6 World Health Organization (WHO) (2002) *Selected Practice Recommendations for Contraceptive Use. Recommendation 10.* WHO, Geneva.
7 Gbolade BA (2002) Depo-Provera and bone density. *Journal of Family Planning and Reproductive Health Care.* **28**(1): 7–11.
8 Mansour D (2001) Contraceptive implants in the United Kingdom. *Contraception Update.* Excerpta Medica.
9 FFPRHC (2003) FFPRHC guidance: emergency contraception. *Journal of Family Planning and Reproductive Health Care.* **29**(2): 9–14.
10 World Health Organization (WHO) (2000) Improving access to quality care in family planning. *Medical Eligibility Criteria for Contraceptive Use.* WHO, Geneva.

Chapter 4

Intrauterine devices

Intrauterine device (IUD)

Legal classification

POM.

Route of administration

Intrauterine.

Efficacy

The intrauterine device (IUD) is 98–100% effective.

IUDs currently available in the UK

Device	Licence (years)
T-Safe 380A	8
Multiload 375*	5
Multiload 250 and 250 short*	5
Nova T200	5
Nova T380	5
Flexi T300	5
GyneFix**	5
(Mirena) LNG IUS	5

*The multiload series of devices was designed to reduce the incidence of expulsion by the addition of plastic fins on the lateral curved arms; this has not been borne out in clinical trials.[1]
**GyneFix
Frameless copper-bearing device, designed to reduce the incidence of bleeding, pain and expulsion seen with framed devices; a knot is embedded in the fundal myometrium and polypropylene threads bear six copper bands. Specialist training to insert is required.[1]

How to use

The IUD needs to be inserted by a trained practitioner. *See* Figure 4.1a–g (Nova T380, reproduced courtesy of Schering Health Care) and 4.2a–g (T-Safe 380A, reproduced courtesy of Eurim-Pharm) for insertion technique.

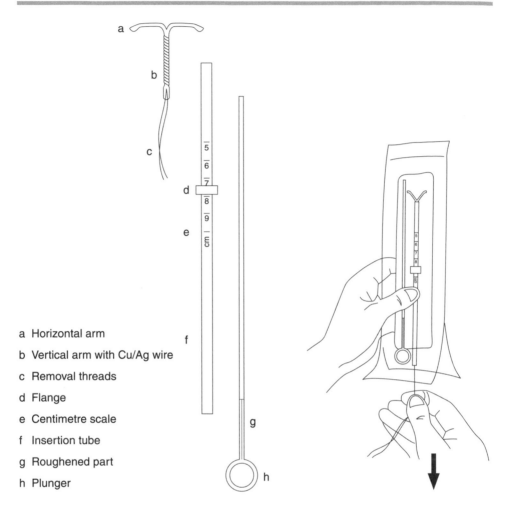

a Horizontal arm

b Vertical arm with Cu/Ag wire

c Removal threads

d Flange

e Centimetre scale

f Insertion tube

g Roughened part

h Plunger

Figure 4.1a   **Figure 4.1b**

How to insert Nova T380

To be inserted by a qualified healthcare professional.

Preinsertion procedure

Make sure that the pouch containing Nova T380 is undamaged before opening it.

- Follow strict asepsis during the insertion.
- Visualise the cervix by means of a speculum and cleanse it with antiseptic solution. Grasp the anterior lip with a tenaculum. A gentle traction on the tenaculum reduces the angle between the cervical canal and the uterine cavity and facilitates introduction of a uterine sound. The tenaculum should remain in position throughout the insertion of Nova T380 to maintain a gentle traction on the cervix.

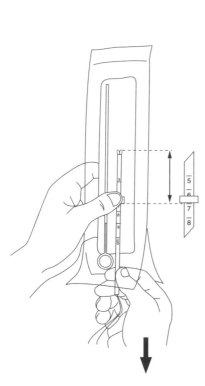

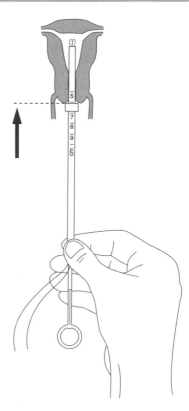

Figure 4.1c **Figure 4.1d**

- Introduce the uterine sound through the cervical canal into the uterine cavity until it reaches the fundus. After determining the direction and length of the cervical canal and the uterine cavity, prepare Nova T380 for insertion.
- Conduct insertion as illustrated in Steps 1–6.

1 After sounding the uterus, open the package halfway.

   Grasp both threads and pull the device gently, not more than 5 minutes prior to the insertion, into the insertion tube until the knobs at the ends of the horizontal arms cover the opening of the tube. The knobs should not be pulled into the tube. Please note that pulling too hard may break the threads.

2 Steadying the yellow flange with one hand, pull the insertion tube until the lower edge of the flange indicates the measure obtained with the uterine sound.

   Holding the threads straight in the tube with one hand, place the plunger into the insertion tube. This ensures that the threads are not pressed against the device by the plunger.

   Prior to insertion, the tube can be bent to conform to the position of the uterus. The bending must be performed whilst the device remains in the sterile package after placing the plunger into the insertion tube.

3 Ensure that the flange indicates the direction in which the horizontal arms will open in the uterus.

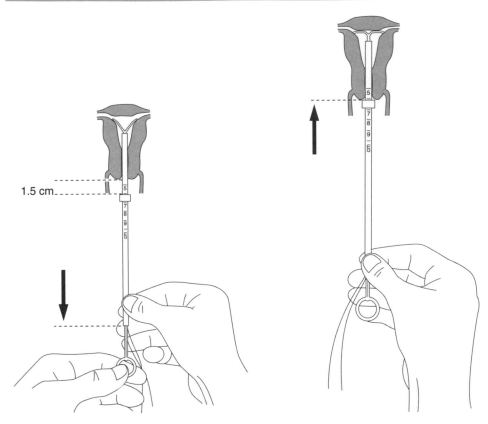

Figure 4.1e   **Figure 4.1f**

Remove the loaded insertion tube from the package.

Introduce the insertion tube through the cervical canal into the uterus until the flange touches the cervical os.

4 Note the roughened part on the plunger. Hold the plunger still and release the horizontal arms of the device by pulling the insertion tube downwards until the edge of the inserter reaches the roughened part.

Observe that the distance between the flange and the cervical os is now about 1.5 cm.

5 Holding the tube and the plunger together, gently push the device until the flange again touches the cervical os.

6 Holding the plunger steady, release the device from the insertion tube completely by pulling the tube down to the ring of the plunger.

To prevent pulling the device from the fundal position, first remove the plunger while keeping the insertion tube steady, and only then remove the insertion tube.

Cut the threads leaving 2–3 cm visible outside the cervix.

Important!

Should you suspect that the device is not in the correct position, remove it and insert a new, sterile device. A removed device must not be re-inserted.

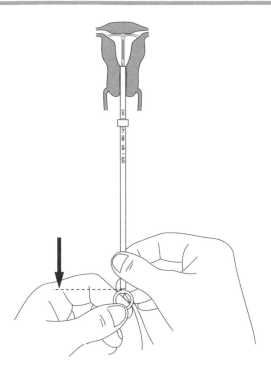

Figure 4.1g

Briefly review the contents of the 'Patient Information' with the patient. Ask the patient to read the information carefully. Fill in the record of insertion in the Patient Information leaflet.

How to insert T-Safe® 380A

The IUD may be used by trained medical staff only. In order to minimise the risk of contamination the use of sterile gloves is recommended.

1 Open the sterile packaging of the T-Safe® CU 200B/380A. Take the loading capsule (a) and push it over the side arms (*see* Figure 4.2a).
2 Push the side arms as far as they will go into the loading capsule until they fit completely in it and pull the insertion tube (b) back carefully until the T-Safe® CU 200B/380A lies freely in the loading capsule (*see* Figure 4.2b).
3 Now squeeze the loading capsule gently on the side and push the insertion tube approximately up to the half over the side arms of the T-Safe® CU 200B. With the T-Safe® CU 380A push the insertion tube up to the end of the copper

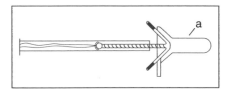

Figure 4.2a

Figure 4.2b

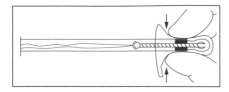

Figure 4.2c

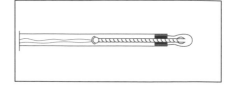

Figure 4.2d

sleeves (*see* Figure 4.2c). The side arms may not be further slid into the insertion tube, since otherwise the tube can be stretched too strongly and unpleasant edges can arise.

4   Remove the loading capsule. T-Safe® CU 200B/380A fits safely in the insertion tube (*see* Figure 4.2d).

5   Holding the threads straight in the tube, place the plunger (c) into the insertion tube. This prevents the threads being disarranged by inserting the plunger.

Adjust the sliding flange (d) so that the length of the tube above it corresponds to the depth of the uterus as previously measured by hysterometry. Ensure that the wider part of the flange indicates the direction in which the side arms of the IUD will open in the uterus (*see* Figure 4.2e).

Note: The ends of the side arms of the T-Safe® 200B/380A must not be slid further into the insertion tube than described under 3 and must not remain bended for over 5 minutes within the insertion tube; otherwise they may not bend back completely and may not return to their original 90° angle.

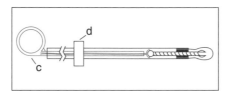

Figure 4.2e

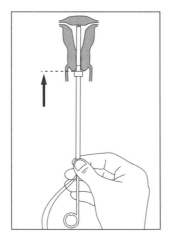

Figure 4.2f

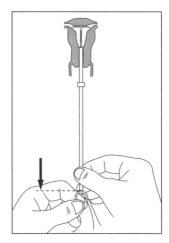

Figure 4.2g

6 Carefully introduce the insertion tube containing the T-Safe® CU 200B/380A into the uterine cavity until it touches the fundus of the uterus. The sliding flange must be in contact with the cervix (*see* Figure 4.2f).

7 Holding the plunger steady, pull the insertion tube downwards to the base of the plunger. The side arms of the IUD are not entirely released in the uterus (*see* Figure 4.2g).

   To prevent pulling the device from its fundal position, first remove the plunger while keeping the insertion tube steady and only then remove the insertion tube.

   Cut the threads leaving 2–3 cm visible outside the cervix.

Removal

T-Safe® CU 200B should be replaced after three years.

T-Safe® CU 380A should be replaced after ten years.

Again, during menstruation is the most appropriate time to remove the IUD, since both the internal and external cervical os are fully dilated. Grasp the threads of the IUD with a tenaculum and pull it along the longitudinal axis of the uterus. Try to insert the forceps at the entrance to the cervical canal in order to grasp the vertical arm of the T-Safe® CU 200B/380A as soon as it has passed the internal cervical os. This avoids excessive tension on the threads which could cause them to break. While doing this, distract the patient's attention by asking her to cough, and then remove the T-Safe® CU 200B/380A with one firm tug.

Insertion and removal of the IUD could cause slight pain and bleeding. The intervention may also precipitate a vasovagal attack or an epileptic seizure.

After removal is complete, inspect the T-Safe® 200B/380A to see that none of its arms have been left in the uterine cavity.

In case of a lost IUD or lost part of an IUD in the uterine cavity either hysteroscopy or ultrasonography or x-rays should be used to determine its location: curettage may be advisable. In very rare cases of uterine perforation laparascopy may be needed.

Pharmacodynamics

The primary mode of action of copper-bearing devices is fertilisation prevention:

- the number of sperm reaching the uterine tubes is reduced
- sperm motility is disrupted
- ova development is impeded.

The prevention of implantation as a result of biochemical and histological changes in the endometrium plays a minor role. Also alterations in the copper content of cervical mucus are seen; this may inhibit sperm penetration.[2]

Indications

An IUD is suitable for women who prefer a longer-term, non-hormonal method of contraception, or where hormones are contraindicated. It is user friendly as it does not involve regular doses, and is most suitable for women who have had a vaginal delivery (although it can be fitted through a nulliparous cervix).

Absolute contraindications

- Pregnancy.
- Suspicion of pregnancy.
- Undiagnosed irregular vaginal bleeding.
- Symptoms suggesting or proven current pelvic infection.
- Distorted/scarred or small uterine cavities.
- Allergy to one of the constituents.
- Wilson's disease.
- Past history of bacterial endocarditis.

Relative contraindications

- Past history of ectopic pregnancy.
- Valvular heart disease (no history of bacterial endocarditis).
- Past history of pelvic infection.
- Lifestyle risking STI.
- Nulliparity and young age.
- Uterine anomalies.
- Menorrhagia or severe primary dysmenorrhoea.

Drug interactions

The available experience with copper-bearing IUDs indicates that drug effects interfering with their contraceptive efficacy are highly unlikely.[3]

Side effects

Bleeding

One of the most common reasons given for the removal of the IUD is bleeding problems. Framed devices can increase menstrual loss by 20–30%.[1] Although IUDs do not affect ovulation, the luteal phase of the cycle is shorter and the onset of menstrual bleeding occurs earlier.[4] Some data suggest that blood loss is less with frameless devices. An IUD may not be the method of first choice for women with excessive menstrual bleeding or anaemia, or for women receiving anticoagulants.[3]

Pain

Associated cramping can occur with an IUD; this symptom occurs less in multiparous clients and women using smaller and frameless devices that do not distort the uterine cavity.[1]

Risks

Pelvic infection

Evidence shows that the presence of IUD threads does not increase the rate of pelvic inflammatory disease (PID) among users of IUDs. The risk of pelvic infection is six times higher during the first 20 days following an IUD insertion than in long-term use. This is thought to be caused by the presence of a pre-existing asymptomatic, cervical STI. Studies have shown that the risk of PID in the month following IUD insertion did not increase significantly, even in the presence of chlamydia, compared to women without infection. Women with gonorrhoea, however, were at an eightfold increased risk of developing PID compared to non-infected women.[5] Selective screening for chlamydia and other STIs prior to insertion may decrease the risk of post-insertion infection.[6]

Advice regarding the importance of seeking prompt advice in the event of excessive pain/vaginal discharge is important as early reporting of symptoms and effective treatment reduces long-term morbidity.

The World Health Organization Medical Eligibility Criteria (WHOMEC) recommends that an IUD should not be inserted when a woman currently has PID or has had it within the last three months.[7]

Actinomyces-like organisms

Actinomyces-like organisms (ALOs) found on routine cervical smears taken from IUD/IUS users is related to the duration of IUD/IUS use and not the type of IUD in place. The incidence of acute infection with ALOs is extremely low, but when it does occur, severe pelvic infection may require treatment by pelvic clearance as a life-saving measure. Asymptomatic women should be counselled with regard to the symptoms of pelvic actinomycoses, the very small risk of developing the disease and management options.

Symptoms of pelvic actinomycoses are:

- intermenstrual bleeding
- pelvic pain
- deep dispareunia
- dysuria.

Clients with ALOs and a copper IUD *in situ* should be monitored every six months for symptoms and have a bimanual examination; alternatively the device can be removed and a new device inserted.[1]

Ectopic pregnancy

Even though ectopic pregnancies may occur when IUDs are used, current data indicate that copper IUD users do not have a higher overall risk of ectopic pregnancy than women using no contraception.[8] However, a pregnancy with an IUD in place is more likely to be ectopic than if pregnancy occurs without an IUD *in situ*. Women with a previous ectopic pregnancy, pelvic surgery or pelvic infection carry a higher risk of ectopic pregnancy. The possibility of ectopic pregnancy should be considered in the case of lower abdominal pain – especially in connection with missed periods or if an amenorrhoeic woman starts bleeding.

Pregnancy

If the woman becomes pregnant when using an IUD, removal of the device is recommended, since the IUD left *in situ* may increase the risk of abortion and preterm labour. Removal of the IUD or probing of the uterus may result in spontaneous abortion. If the device cannot be gently removed, termination of the pregnancy may be considered. If the woman wishes to continue the pregnancy and the device cannot be withdrawn, she should be informed about these risks and the possible consequence of premature birth to the infant. In addition, ectopic pregnancy should be excluded and the course of such a pregnancy should be closely monitored. The woman should be instructed to report all symptoms that suggest complications of the pregnancy, like cramping abdominal pain with fever. She should be informed that, to date, there is no evidence of birth defects in cases where a pregnancy continues to term with the IUD in place.[1]

Perforation

Uterine perforation at the time of IUD insertion is rare. Failure to stabilise the cervix at insertion and to ascertain the uterine size and position can lead to perforation. Perforations also tend to be more common early in the postpartum period, particularly if the woman is breastfeeding.[9]

A uterine perforation may be diagnosed at the time of insertion; the IUD can then be easily removed with no other action necessary. However, a perforation may also be silent and only recognised when the thread of the IUD cannot be felt at subsequent examination or when the woman becomes pregnant. If a perforation is suspected then the device should be located by ultrasound or radiograph and removed by laparoscopy or laparotomy.

Expulsion

Expulsion can occur at any time after insertion, but the most common time is at the first post-insertion menses. About 20% of expulsions are detected by the client; it often goes unnoticed and can account for one-third of the pregnancies associated with IUD use.[1]

Advice to clients

Insertion

- A copper IUD can be inserted up to five days following the earliest estimated time of ovulation (i.e. before implantation). This is particularly useful when multiple episodes of unprotected sexual intercourse have occurred during a cycle.
- Immediately after TOP or miscarriage, the risk of expulsion following a second-trimester abortion is higher; however, the benefits of IUD insertion still outweigh the risks.[7]

- Early insertion postpartum is also safe, after four weeks. WHOMEC suggests an increased risk of perforation if an IUD is inserted between 48 hours and four weeks postpartum.[7]

Removal

It is advisable to remove the IUD at the time of a period; it will be easier at this time and will also reduce the chance of an iatrogenic pregnancy. If removed at any other time and pregnancy is not desired, advice to avoid sexual intercourse for seven days before removal is recommended.

Intrauterine system (IUS)

Legal classification

POM.

Route of administration

Intrauterine.

Efficacy

The intrauterine system (IUS) is 99–100% effective.

Formulations

Mirena (*see* Figure 4.3a–m, reproduced courtesy of Schering Health)
   The Mirena is a T-shaped plastic frame (impregnated with barium sulphate and with threads attached to the base) with a polydimethylsiloxan reservoir releasing 20 mcg of levonorgestrel (LNG) every 24 hours for five years.

How to use

The IUS is inserted into the uterine cavity by a trained professional.

How to insert Mirena® (Schering Health)

To be inserted by a healthcare professional.
   Mirena® is supplied sterile. Mirena® is sterilised with ethylene oxide. Do not resterilise. For single use only. Do not use if the inner package is damaged or open. Insert before the month shown on the label.
   Mirena® is inserted with the provided inserter (Figure 4.3a) into the uterine cavity within 7 days of the onset of menstruation by carefully following the insertion instructions.
   It can be replaced by a new system at any time of the cycle.

Preparation for insertion

- Examine the woman to establish the size and position of the uterus to detect acute cervicitis or other contraindications and to exclude pregnancy.
- Make sure that the insertion technique will be aseptic. Use appropriate antiseptic solution to clean the vagina.
- Visualise the cervix by means of a speculum and thoroughly cleanse the cervix and vagina with a suitable antiseptic solution.
- Use assistance as necessary.
- Grasp the upper lip of the cervix with holding forceps. Gentle traction on the holding forceps has been shown to straighten the cervical canal. The forceps should remain in position throughout the insertion procedure to maintain gentle traction on the cervix against the pushing force of the insertion.
- Gently move a uterine sound across the uterine cavity to the fundus to determine the direction of the cervical canal and the depth of the uterine cavity (sound measure) and to exclude a uterine septum, synechiae and submucous fibroids. Should the cervical canal be too narrow, dilation of the canal is recommended. Consider the use of analgesics/paracervical block.

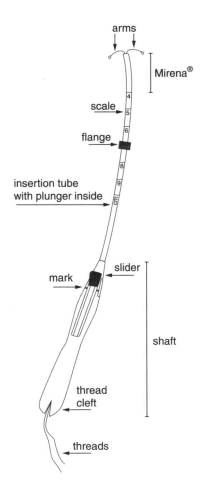

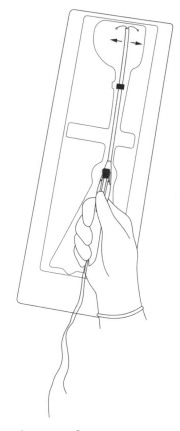

Figure 4.3a   **Figure 4.3b**

Insertion

1 First open the sterile package. Then using sterile gloves, release the threads. Make sure that the slider is in the furthest position away from operator (nearest the cervical end).

   Grab the shaft and check that the arms of the system are in a horizontal position (shape of T). If they are not, align them on a sterile surface (Figure 4.3b).

2 Pull on the threads (Figure 4.3c) to place the Mirena® system in the insertion tube.

   - Note that the knobs at the ends of the arms now close the open end of the inserter (Figure 4.3d). Ensure that the arms will fold out horizontally. If not, open the arms by pulling the slider further back to the mark (Figure 4.3e).
   - Align the open arms on a sterile surface as shown in Figure 4.3b.
   - Return the slider into its furthermost position and hold it firmly with your forefinger or thumb.

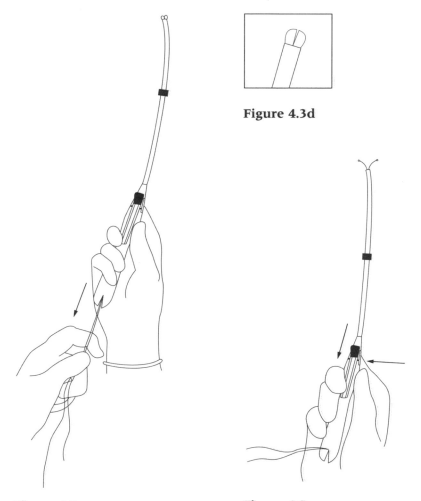

Figure 4.3d

Figure 4.3c   **Figure 4.3e**

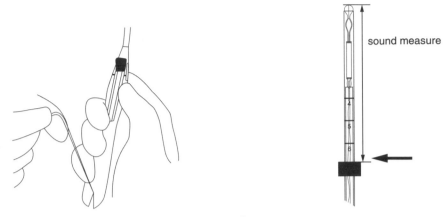

Figure 4.3f   **Figure 4.3g**

3 Fix the threads tightly in the cleft at the near end of the inserter shaft (Figure 4.3f).
4 Set the flange to the sound measurement as indicated in Figure 4.3g.
5 Mirena® is now ready to be inserted.
   Hold the slider with your forefinger or thumb firmly in the further-most position. Move the inserter carefully through the cervical canal into the uterus until the flange is situated at a distance of about 1.5–2 cm from the cervix to give sufficient space for the arms to open (Figure 4.3h).
   Note! Do not force the inserter.
6 While holding the inserter steady release the arms of Mirena® (Figure 4.3i) by pulling the slider back until it reaches the mark (Figure 4.3j).
7 Push the inserter gently inwards until the flange touches the cervix. Mirena® should now be in the fundal position (Figure 4.3k).
8 Holding the inserter firmly in position release Mirena® by pulling down the slider all the way. The threads will straighten out automatically (Figure 4.3l).

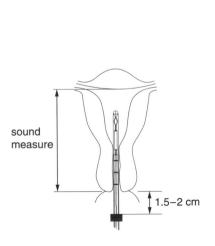

Figure 4.3h

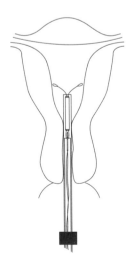

Figure 4.3i

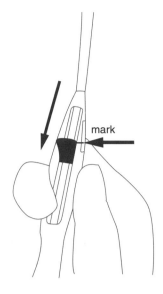

Figure 4.3j

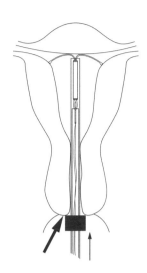

Figure 4.3k

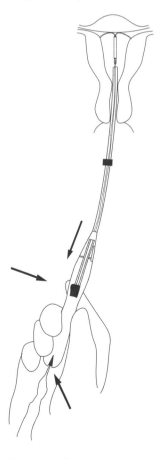

Figure 4.3l

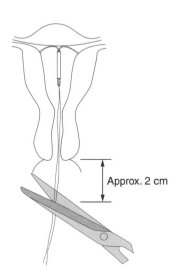

Figure 4.3m

9 Remove the inserter from the uterus. Cut the threads to leave about 2 cm visible outside the cervix (Figure 4.3m).

Important!

Should you suspect that the system is not in the correct position, check, e.g. with ultrasound and if necessary remove the system and insert a new, sterile system. A removed system must not be re-inserted.

Removal of Mirena®

Mirena® can be removed by pulling the threads with forceps.

Special notes

In order to maintain reliable contraception the system should not be removed after the fifth day of the menstrual cycle. Otherwise contraception has to be ensured with other methods (e.g. condoms) starting at least 5 days before the removal. When the woman has no menses, she should also use barrier methods of contraception starting 5 days before removal and has to continue with this until her menstruation reappears.

A new Mirena® can also be inserted immediately following removal, in which case no additional protection is needed.

Pharmacodynamics

The IUS works primarily by:

- causing endometrial suppression (this is the main contraceptive effect)
- changing cervical mucus and utero-tubal fluids which impair sperm migration.

Anovulation occurs in some women during the first year of use.[10]

Intrauterine concentrations of LNG are high and as a result:

- endometrial oestrogen and progesterone receptors are downregulated
- there is endometrial atrophy
- there are changes in the endometrial stroma
- there is an increase in inflammatory cell numbers.

This leads to the prevention of implantation.

The IUS has minimal effect on the hypothalamo-pituitary-ovarian axis. Serum oestradiol levels are greater than 100 pg/ml in most women, indicating follicular development. Most women (more than 75%) will continue to ovulate.[10]

Indications

- Client's choice.
- Dysmenorrhoea.

- Menorrhagia: the IUS is the most effective pharmacological treatment for menorrhagia. Incidentally women using the IUS for menorrhagia only, and whose symptoms are well controlled, may continue with the IUS beyond its licensed duration.[3]

Contraindications

- Heart valve replacement or previous history of bacterial endocarditis (increased risk of infection).
- Congenital or acquired uterine anomaly.
- Suspected or confirmed uterine or cervical malignancy.
- Recent trophoblastic disease.
- Severe side effects with the COC not due to oestrogen.
- Current DVT/pulmonary embolus.
- Ischaemic heart disease.
- Active viral hepatitis.
- Severe decompensated cirrhosis.
- Benign liver tumours.
- Malignant hepatoma.

Relative contraindications

- Chronic systemic disease.
- Risk factors for arterial disease.
- Current breast cancer/history of breast cancer in the past five years.
- Functional ovarian cysts that have required hospitalisation.

Breastfeeding

Observational studies have shown low concentrations of LNG in breast milk following insertion of an IUS releasing 10 or 30 mg LNG per day. The use of the IUS by women who are breastfeeding does not appear to have any detrimental effect on infant development.[11]

Drug interactions

- No reduction in the efficacy of the IUS has been identified with liver enzyme inducers.
- No other drugs are known to interact with the IUS.

Side effects

The release of LNG from the IUS is 20 mcg/24 hours, delivered directly into the uterine cavity; because of the low plasma concentrations, there are only minor effects on the metabolism.

A systematic review identified no significant differences in overall side effects (e.g. acne, headaches, breast tenderness, nausea, prolonged bleeding) between women using the IUS or an IUD.[12] Serum LNG levels with the IUS are lower than with oral or subdermal administration but wide interindividual variation in serum LNG occurs; this may explain why there are wide variations in experience of hormonal symptoms.

Reduced bleeding/amenorrhoea

Intrauterine release of levonorgestrel has a local effect on the endometrium, rendering it suppressed and insensitive to oestradiol, resulting in a progressive reduction in the volume and duration of menstruation.

However, the IUS can cause irregular bleeding, particularly in the first three months. Prolonged bleeding (more than eight days) in the first month of use is experienced by 20% of users. The duration and amount of bleeding generally falls during IUS use, with 17% of women experiencing amenorrhoea of at least three months' duration or more in the first year.[12]

The mechanisms underlying bleeding patterns with the IUS are unclear. It suppresses spiral arteriole formation and has a localised effect on some vessels within the endometrium. Matrix metalloproteinases, a family of enzymes within the endometrium, are involved in endometrial breakdown during normal menstruation. Expression of metalloproteinase-9 is increased in the endometrium from IUS users, which may contribute to abnormal bleeding.

The IUS may also help prevent or regulate fibroid growth.

Ectopic pregnancy

WHOMEC recommends that women who have previously had an ectopic pregnancy may use the IUS. Recent studies have shown that the risk of ectopic pregnancy with the IUS is low.[13] The rate of ectopic pregnancy in IUS users is 0.06 per 100 woman-years. This rate is lower than the rate of 0.3–0.5 per 100 woman-years estimated for women not using any contraception.[3]

Ovarian cysts

Some studies have found that there is an increased risk of ovarian cysts with IUS use; however, the majority of cysts were asymptomatic and resolved spontaneously.[14] Case reports suggest that ovarian pathology should be considered in the differential diagnosis of IUS users who present with abdominal pain.[10]

Perforation

The rate of perforation reported with the IUS in a large observational cohort study was 0.9 per 1000 insertions.[15]

Expulsion

Most contraceptive failures with the IUS are due to expulsion. Expulsion rate is 4.5 per 100 users at 12 months, 5.2 at 24 months and 5.9 at 60 months. IUS users are more likely to experience an expulsion than IUD users.[11]

Infection

There is a small increase in the risk of pelvic infection in the 20 days following insertion; thereafter the risk is the same as for the non-IUS-using population. The IUS may limit the risk of pelvic infection by thickening the cervical mucus.

Return of fertility

Studies have shown a pregnancy rate of 90 per 100 women in the first year after IUS removal. The mean time to pregnancy was four months.[16]

Advice to clients

Insertion

- It is recommended that the IUS is inserted within the first seven days of the menstrual cycle, but not during the days of heaviest blood loss when expulsion is more likely. No further extra contraceptive precautions are necessary.
- If a copper IUD is already in place or the woman is taking a hormonal method of contraception, insertion can take place at any time during the cycle (although when replacing an IUD it must be borne in mind that it may not be possible to fit the IUS – therefore pregnancy risk should be taken into consideration).
- Immediate insertion after TOP or miscarriage.
- Six to eight weeks postnatally to reduce the incidence of problematic prolonged bleeding.
- Should not be fitted as a method of postcoital contraception.

Removal

It is advisable to remove the IUS at the time of a period (if the client is having them), as it will be easier at this time and will also reduce the chance of an iatrogenic pregnancy. If removed at any other time and pregnancy is not desired, advice to avoid sexual intercourse for seven days before removal is recommended.

NB: As for Implanon insertion, IUD/IUS insertion requires official theoretical training and specialised training from a Faculty of Family Planning approved teaching doctor; for nurses the RCN has a specific proforma to complete before sending a certificate of competence.

Long-acting reversible contraceptives

The IUD, IUS, contraceptive implant and injection form a group of contraceptive methods that have recently been labelled as 'long-acting reversible contraceptives'. The National Institute for Health and Clinical Excellence has recently issued recommendations that these methods be promoted as a means to reduce unplanned pregnancy and increase cost effectiveness, and it stresses the safety of these methods.

www.nice.org.uk/pdf/cg030niceguidelines.pdf

References

1 Mansour D (2001) Intrauterine contraceptive devices and systems. *Contraception Update*. Excerpta Medica.

2 Ortiz ME and Croxatto MB (1987) The mode of action of IUDs. *Contraception*. **36**: 37–53.

3 Electronic Medicines Compendium: www.emc.medicines.org.uk

4 Faundes A, Segal SJ, Adejuwon CA *et al.* (1980) The menstrual cycle in women using an intrauterine device. *Fertility and Sterility*. **34**: 427–30.

5 Sinei SKA, Schultz KF, Lamptey PR *et al.* (1990) Preventing IUCD related pelvic infection: the efficacy of prophylactic doxycycline at insertion. *British Journal of Obstetrics and Gynaecology*. **97**: 412–19.

6 Faculty of Family Planning and Reproductive Health Care of the Royal College of Obstetricians and Gynaecologists (2002) IUDs: which device? *Journal of Family Planning and Reproductive Health Care*. **28**(2): 1–9.

7 Faculty of Family Planning and Reproductive Health Care Clinical Effectiveness Unit (2004) Guidance: the copper intrauterine device as long-term contraception. *Journal of Family Planning and Reproductive Health Care*. **30**(1): 29–42.

8 Xiong X, Buekens P and Wollast E (1995) IUD use and the risk of ectopic pregnancy: a meta analysis of case-control studies. *Contraception*. **52**: 23–34.

9 World Health Organization (WHO) (2002) *Medical Eligibility Criteria for Contraceptive Use*. WHO, Geneva.

10 Faculty of Family Planning and Reproductive Health Care Clinical Effectiveness Unit (2004) Guidance: the levonorgestrel-releasing intrauterine system in contraception and reproductive health. *Journal of Family Planning and Reproductive Health Care*. **30**(2): 99–108.

11 French RS, Cowan FM, Mansour DJA *et al.* (2000) Implantable contraceptives (subdermal implants and hormonally impregnated intrauterine systems) versus other forms of reversible contraceptives: two systematic reviews to assess relative effectiveness, acceptability, tolerability and cost effectiveness (review). *Health Technology Assessment*. **4**: I–iv, 1–107.

12 Irvine GA, Campbell Brown MB, Lumsden MA *et al.* (1998) Randomised comparative trial of the levenorgestrel intrauterine system and norethisterone for treatment of idiopathic menorrhagia. *British Journal of Obstetrics and Gynaecology*. **90**: 257–63.

13 Sivin I and Stern J (1994) Health during prolonged use of levenorgestrel 20 mg/d and the copper Tcu 380Ag intrauterine contraceptive devices: a multicenter study. *Fertility and Sterility*. **61**: 70–7.

14 Inki P, Hurskainen R, Palo P *et al.* (2002) Comparison of ovarian cyst formation in women using the levonorgestrel-releasing intrauterine system vs hysterectomy. *Ultrasound Obstetrics and Gynaecology*. **20**: 381–5.

15 Zhou L, Harrison Woolrych M and Coulter DM (2003) Use of the New Zealand Intensive Medicines Monitoring Programme to study the levonorgestrel-releasing intrauterine device (Mirena). *Pharmacoepidemiological Drug Safety*. **1**: 371–7.

16 Belhaj H, Sivin I, Diaz S *et al.* (1986) Recovery of fertility after use of the levenorgestrel 20 mcg/d or copper T380 Ag intrauterine device. *Contraception*. **34**: 261–7.

Chapter 5

Spermicides

Spermicidal contraceptives

Legal classification

Pharmacy (P).

Route of administration

Per vagina.

Efficacy

Not applicable.

Formulations

Delfen (Janssen-Cilag)
Foam nonoxynol 9 12.5% pressurised aerosol unit in a water-miscible basis

Duragel (SSL)
Gel nonoxynol 9 2% in a water-soluble basis

Gynol II (Janssen-Cilag)
Jelly nonoxynol 9 2% in a water-soluble basis

Ortho-crème (Janssen-Cilag)
Cream nonoxynol 9 2% in a water-miscible basis

Orthoforms (Janssen-Cilag)
Pessaries nonoxynol 9 5% in a water-soluble basis

Nonoxynol 9 is the only licensed spermicide in the UK.

How to use

Nonoxynol 9 when used alone is moderately effective as a contraceptive.

For women who choose to use nonoxynol 9 alone in preference to other methods it is better than no contraceptive method at all.

However, it is preferable to use spermicide in conjunction with a barrier contraceptive method such as the cervical cap or diaphragm, condom or Femidom. When used with a female mechanical barrier method (i.e. cervical cap or diaphragm), nonoxynol 9 is more effective than when used alone.

Nonoxynol 9 is available in a number of different formulations and doses. It is not known whether contraceptive effectiveness differs according to formulation or dose.

Pharmacodynamics

Spermicides have two main components: a relatively inert base and an active spermicidal agent. Hence they operate both physically and biochemically, forming a partial barrier and also immobilising sperm.

The main site of action of nonoxynol 9 has been determined as the sperm cell membrane. The lipoprotein membrane is disrupted, increasing permeability, with subsequent loss of cell components and decreased motility. A similar effect on vaginal epithelial and bacterial cells is also found.[1]

Advantages

- Suitable for women looking for an easily available method.
- No major health risks associated with spermicide use.
- Only need be used with or immediately prior to sexual intercourse (at least ten minutes and no longer than one hour before).
- Provides lubrication.

Disadvantages

- Not suitable for women looking for a highly effective contraceptive method.
- May cause local irritation.
- Potentially increased possibility of STI transmission with increased use.

Drug interactions

None known.

Side effects

- Increasing frequency of nonoxynol 9 use increases the risk of epithelial disruption.
- There is good evidence that nonoxynol 9 does not reduce the risk of STIs or HIV among sex workers, nor among women attending STI clinics. In fact high-frequency use and higher doses of nonoxynol 9 products may cause epithelial damage and increase the risk of HIV infection. The spermicide causes some degree of epithelial disruption and may alter the vaginal microflora; they thus have the potential to increase penetration by infectious elements.

Condoms and nonoxynol 9

There is no published scientific evidence that nonoxynol 9 lubricated condoms provide any additional protection against pregnancy or STIs compared with condoms lubricated with other products (*see* side effects). Since adverse effects due to the addition of nonoxynol 9 to condoms cannot be excluded, such condoms should no longer be promoted.[2]

References

1   Electronic Medicines Compendium: www.emc.medicines.org.uk
2   World Health Organization (WHO) (2001) *Nonoxynol 9*. WHO, Geneva.

Chapter 6

Barrier methods

Diaphragms and caps

Legal classification

POM.

Route of administration

Per vagina.

Efficacy

The diaphragm and cap are 92% to 96% effective.

Contraceptive caps

Type A contraceptive pessary

Opaque rubber, sizes 1–5 (55–75 mm rising in steps of 5 mm). Available from Lamberts (Dumas Vault Cap).

Type B contraceptive pessary

Opaque rubber, sizes 22–31 mm (rising in steps of 3 mm). Available from Lamberts (Prentif Cavity Rim Cervical Cap).

Type C contraceptive pessary

Opaque rubber, sizes 1–3 (42, 48 and 54 mm). Available from Lamberts (Vimule cap).

Cervical cap

Shaped like a thimble and designed to fit snugly over the cervix.

Vault cap

Bowl shaped; covers but does not fit closely to the cervix.

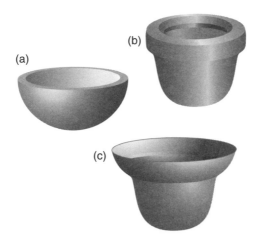

Figure 6.1 (a) Vault cap; (b) cervical cap; (c) vimule cap.

Vimule

A variation of the vault cap with a hat-shaped prolongation of the dome to accommodate longer cervicies.

See Figure 6.1.

Contraceptive diaphragms

Type A diaphragm with flat metal spring

Transparent rubber with flat metal spring, sizes 55–95 mm (rising in steps of 5 mm).
Available from Janssen-Cilag (Reflexions).

Type B diaphragm with coiled metal rim

Opaque rubber with coiled metal rim, sizes 60–100 mm (rising in steps of 5 mm).
Available from Janssen-Cilag (Ortho).

Type C arching-spring diaphragm

Opaque rubber with arching spring, sizes 60–95 mm (rising in steps of 5 mm).
Available from Janssen-Cilag (All-Flex).

Flat-spring diaphragm

Firm spring and is easily fitted; suitable for the normal vagina and is often tried first.

Coil-spring diaphragm

Spiral coiled spring; softer than the flat spring.

Arching-spring diaphragm

Combines features of both the above; firm double metal spring. Exerts strong pressure on the vaginal walls.

How to use

Cap

Caps work by suction and act as a barrier to sperm.

- Prevents cervical mucus entering the vagina.
- Prevents physical aspiration of sperm into the cervix and uterus.

How to fit a cap
- The correct size of cap allows the rim of the cap to touch the fornices with no gap, accommodating the cervix and showing evidence of a suction effect.

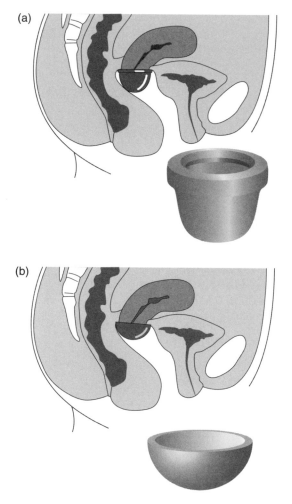

Figure 6.2   Correct positioning of (a) cervical cap; (b) vault cap.

- To insert, the rim is compressed between thumb and fingers and guided along the posterior vaginal wall towards the cervix. The cap is then allowed to open and is pushed over the cervix with the fingertips.
- To remove the cap, insert a fingertip above the rim and then ease it downwards.
- Once the instructor has fitted the device for the client, the client should then feel for her cervix through the device to know the correct positioning.
- During the fitting the client can then remove the device and re-insert it herself; this can be tricky at first but will become easier with practice.

See Figure 6.2 for the correct positioning of a cap.

Diaphragm

- Acts as a carrier of spermicide.
- Holds sperm away from cervical mucus long enough for them to die in the acidic vagina.
- Prevents cervical mucus entering the vagina.
- Prevents physical aspiration of sperm into the cervix and uterus.

How to fit a diaphragm

- Assess the size of diaphragm required by measuring the distance from the posterior fornix (the area immediately behind the cervix) to the symphysis pubis (the bone in front of the bladder) with your fingers. The measurement on your fingers corresponds to the size of the diaphragm required for your client. *See* Figure 6.3.
- Fold the diaphragm in half by pressing opposite sides together.
- The diaphragm is inserted into the vagina downwards and backwards to the posterior fornix, tucking the anterior rim behind the symphysis pubis.
- Check the cervix is covered. *See* Figure 6.4.
- On fitting insert a fingertip between the anterior rim of the cap and the symphysis; if the diaphragm is too small a wider gap will be felt or that

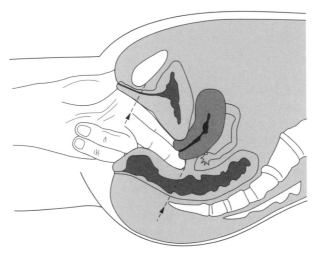

Figure 6.3   Diaphragm: assessing the size.

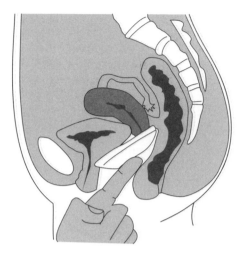

Figure 6.4 Diaphragm: check the cervix is covered.

the whole diaphragm is in the anterior fornix; if the diaphragm is too large it projects inferiorly/anteriorly and may cause immediate discomfort or become uncomfortable later. *See* Figures 6.5a, b.
- Once the instructor has fitted the device for the client, the client should then feel for her cervix through the device to know the correct positioning.
- During the fitting the client can then remove the device and re-insert it herself; this can be tricky at first but will become easier with practice.

It is useful to demonstrate the insertion and positioning of a diaphragm/cap on a plastic model so the client can picture its positioning in her body.

Pharmacodynamics

The cap and diaphragm are physical barriers to sperm penetration.

Advantages

- Effective if used with care.
- Women in control of use, and needs only be used when required.
- Aesthetically useful for intercourse during uterine bleeding.
- No proven systemic effects.
- Offers some protection against most STIs, including the agents causing PID, by providing a mechanical barrier which reduces the chance of organisms reaching the cervix and upper genital tract. This will not be enough protection against viruses, including herpes or non-viral diseases like syphilis, which can form lesions of the vagina, vulva and elsewhere.
- Reduction in risk of cervical neoplasia – in the Oxford/fpa study the rate per 100 women-years for oral contraceptive users was 0.95 and for IUD users 0.87. For diaphragm users the rate was 0.23 after adjustment for age at first coitus, number of partners and smoking patterns.[1]

(a)

(b)

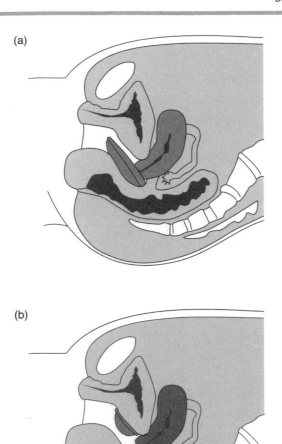

Figure 6.5 Incorrect fitting of the diaphragm: (a) diaphragm too large; (b) diaphragm too small.

Disadvantages

- Involves a women handling her own genitalia, some forward planning, some loss of spontaneity.
- Requires fitting by trained professional.
- Less effective than hormonal contraception or IUD.
- Sometimes perceived as being messy.
- Can produce some local adverse effects:
  - increased risk of urinary tract infection (less so for caps) – the fact that urinary tract infections (UTIs) develop more frequently is believed to be caused mainly by the pressure of the rim on the urethra and bladder base, predisposing to urethritis and cystitis

– vaginal irritation and/or allergy due to rubber or spermicide
– pressure from rim can cause, rarely, vaginal abrasions or ulcers.
- Some studies have suggested that diaphragm and cap use with spermicide can alter the vaginal flora so as to promote infections.[2]

Common reasons for failure

User

- Failure to use.
- Failure to check that the cervix is covered.

Clinician

- Wrong selection of users.
- Poor fitting.
- Poor teaching.

Contraindications

- Aversion to touching the genital area.
- Congenital abnormalities such as septate vagina.
- Uterovaginal prolapse.
- Poor vaginal or perineal muscle tone.
- Inability to learn the insertion technique.
- Recurrent UTIs (could use vault or cervical cap).
- Rubber allergy.
- Pregnancy.
- Undiagnosed genital tract bleeding.
- Current infection.
- Past history of toxic shock syndrome.

Drug interactions

As for nonoxynol 9 (used in conjuction with diaphragm or cap). Preparations that could perish the devices' rubber should not be used, e.g. baby oil, body oil etc.

Side effects/risks

See Disadvantages.

Advice to clients

The best positions to insert and check a diaphragm or cap are standing with one foot on a chair or squatting.

Spermicide

Cap

Spermicide should fill one-third of the bowl. None should be put on the rim so as not to impair suction. An extra measure of spermicidal jelly or pessary should be added on the vaginal side before the first as well as subsequent sexual intercourse after insertion.

Diaphragm

For use prior to sexual intercourse: two strips of spermicide should be applied to both sides of the diaphragm; some spermicide can be put on the rim to aid insertion.

Duration of use

Diaphragm and cap

Leave the device in for at least six hours after sexual intercourse. If more than three hours elapses after insertion and sexual intercourse you will need to insert additional spermicide. If additional episodes of sex occur before the six hours has elapsed more spermicide will be required and the diaphragm not removed until six hours after the last sexual intercourse.

The cap or diaphragm should be washed in warm water with mild soap; it should be thoroughly dried and stored in its box in a cool, dry place.

If there is weight change by 3 kg (either loss or gain) the client will need refitting as vaginal dimensions may have also changed.

Condoms

How to use

The condom is put over an erect penis to catch sperm and prevent it entering the vagina.

Condoms come in different varieties. They can be different flavours, colours, ribbed, be made of latex or polyurethane and be sensitive or extra strong.

Condoms can be either spermicidally or non-spermicidally lubricated. *See* Chapter 5 on spermicides regarding recommendations for use.

See Figure 6.6 overleaf for how to use a condom.

Pharmacodynamics

Condoms act as a physical barrier to sperm entering the vagina.

Indications

As well as stopping pregnancy, condoms are the only method that also protect against STIs; they are recommended for use where there is a risk of contracting an STI from vaginal, anal and oral sexual intercourse.

Step 1	Check for (CE) mark – the European standard mark (indication of quality standard; has been tested). Check the condom is in date. Check for tears and rips in the packet. Any hole in the packet will mean the condom has dried out and may split. It is best to keep condoms in a dry, cool place. Put the condom on when the penis is erect, before there is any contact between the penis and the partner's body. Fluid released from the penis during the early stages of an erection (pre-ejaculate) can contain sperm.
Step 2 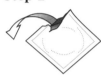	Push the condom down to the bottom of the packet and carefully tear along one side of the foil, being sure not to rip the condom inside. Teeth and nails can make a hole in the condom. Carefully remove the condom.
Step 3 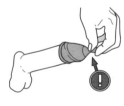	Air trapped inside a condom can cause it to break. To avoid this, squeeze the closed end of the condom between your forefinger and thumb and place the condom over the erect penis. Be sure that the roll is on the outside. If you find the condom is on upside down and isn't rolling, throw it away and start again. If you just turn it around there will be sperm on the outside from the pre-ejaculate.
Step 4 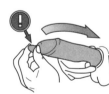	While still squeezing the closed end, use your other hand to unroll the condom gently down the full length of the penis.
Step 5 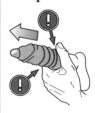	Soon after ejaculation, withdraw the penis while it is still erect by holding the condom firmly in place. Remove the condom only when the penis is fully withdrawn. Keep both the penis and condom clear from contact with your partner's body.

Figure 6.6 How to use a condom.

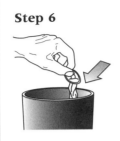

| Step 6 | Dispose of the used condom hygienically. Wrap it in a tissue and place it in a bin. (Do not flush it down the toilet.) |

Figure 6.6   *(continued)*

Disadvantages

- Condom use must be negotiated between both partners.
- May be seen as interrupting sex.
- Can burst, split or slip during sexual intercourse.
- Allergy to the condom.
- Loss of sensation.

Contraindications

Allergy to latex or spermicide.

Female condom: Femidom

How to use

Femidom is a prelubricated, soft, polyurethane sheath that lines the vagina and acts as a barrier to sperm entering the vagina. There is a smaller inner ring and larger outer ring. The smaller inner ring is used to feed the Femidom into the vagina. Most of the Femidom goes inside the woman and the larger ring overlaps the outer area of the vagina.

See Figure 6.7 overleaf for how to use a Femidom.

Pharmacodynamics

The Femidom acts as a physical barrier to sperm entering the vagina.

Indications

- As well as stopping pregnancy, Femidoms also protect against STIs; they are recommended for use where there is a risk of contracting an STI from vaginal sexual intercourse.
- Femidoms can also be used for anal intercourse, though there is no scientific basis for this.

Continued on p. 84

Step 1

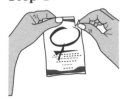

Open the package carefully; tear at the notch on the top right of the package. Do not use scissors or a knife to open.

Step 2

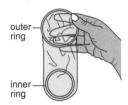

outer ring

inner ring

The outer ring covers the area around the opening of the vagina. The inner ring is used for insertion and to help hold the sheath in place during intercourse.

Step 3

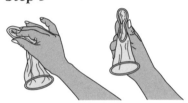

While holding the sheath at the closed end, grasp the flexible inner ring and squeeze it with the thumb and second or middle finger so it becomes long and narrow.

Step 4

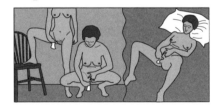

Choose a position that is comfortable for insertion – squat, raise one leg, sit or lie down.

Step 5

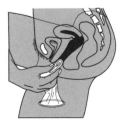

Gently insert the inner ring into the vagina. Feel the inner ring go up and move into place.

Figure 6.7 How to use a femidom.

Step 6 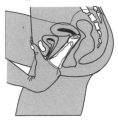	Place the index finger on the inside of the condom and push the inner ring up as far as it will go. Be sure the sheath is not twisted. The outer ring should remain on the outside of the vagina.
Step 7 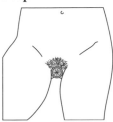	The female condom is now in place and ready for use with your partner.
Step 8 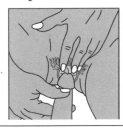	When you are ready, gently guide your partner's penis into the sheath's opening with your hand to make sure that it enters properly – be sure that the penis is not entering on the side, between the sheath and the vaginal wall.
Step 9 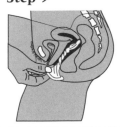	To remove the condom, twist the outer ring and gently pull the condom out.
Step 10 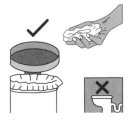	Dispose of the used condom hygienically. Wrap it in the package or in tissue and throw it in the bin. (Do not flush it down the toilet.)

Figure 6.7   (*continued*)

- In some countries Femidoms are re-used. Again this is not a recommended use, although the World Health Organization recognises that it is better to use a used Femidom rather than no protection.[3]

Advantages

- The woman has control over use.
- It protects against STIs.

Disadvantages

- Some people find them noisy.
- May be seen as interrupting sex.

Contraindications

Allergy to spermicide.

Oral shields (dental dams) (non-contraceptive)

How to use

Oral shields are small sheets of latex. They are used as a barrier during oral sex (vaginal or anal) and can protect against STIs. Oral shields should be used once only.

Simply place the oral shield over the vulva – the female sexual organs, including the clitoris, vagina and labia – or over the anus for rimming. It's a good idea to use some water-based lubricant between the shield and your partner's vulva or anus for added sensation.

In order to avoid cross-infection, it is advisable that each partner uses their own oral shield. It is also advisable to mark one side of the shield in order to highlight which side has been used.

Pharmacodynamics

Acts as a barrier to the transmission of STIs.

Indications

A six-inch square of pure latex that can be used to make oral sex (vaginal or anal) safer for women and men. It is called a dental dam because it was originally used for patient protection in dentistry.

Contraindications

Allergy to latex.

References

1 Guillebaud J (2004) *Contraception Today*. Martin Dunitz. London.
2 Everett S (2004) *Handbook of Contraception and Reproductive Sexual Health* (2e). Ballière Tindall, London.
3 Smith EJ (2003) Female condom reuse: issues explored. *Network*. **22**(4). www.fhi.org/en/RH/Pubs/Network/v22_4/index.htm

Chapter 7

Contraceptive options after childbirth

	When to use/fit postpartum	Use with breastfeeding	Failure rate (first-year failure rates per 100 women)	Additional notes
Combined oral contraceptive pills/patch	Day 21	No	0.1–3	In breastfeeding women a COC is not recommended before six weeks postpartum. It can be considered after six weeks if all other contraceptive methods are unacceptable.
Progestogen-only pills	Up to day 21	Yes	0.3–4	Needs to be taken regularly. May result in irregular bleeding although this is more acceptable/less problematic in breastfeeding women.
Contraceptive injection	Usually six weeks	Yes	0–1	Injections are effective for 12 weeks. If given soon after giving birth can cause heavy/irregular bleeding. Fertility may not return for several months after stopping injections.
Implant	From day 21 to 28	Yes	0–0.7	Effective for three years. May cause irregular bleeding.
Intrauterine system	From four weeks postpartum	Yes	0.1–0.2	Effective for up to five years. After about three months, periods usually become much lighter and shorter. Local delivery also minimises side effects. Following fitting from day 28 onwards, extra precautions required for seven days.

Copper intrauterine device	Fit immediately or delay to four weeks postpartum	Yes	0.2–1	Effective for three to eight years depending on type used. May cause periods to be heavier, longer or more painful.
Natural methods	Ask family planning adviser	Yes	2–25	More difficult to do just after childbirth as fertility signs are harder to interpret. Persona cannot be used after recent childbirth or if breastfeeding.*
Lactational amenorrhoea**	Immediately postpartum	Yes	0–2	Only effective before periods return and when fully breastfeeding a baby under six months, e.g. every two to four hours. Not effective if using a combination of bottle and breastfeeding.
Diaphragm	Six weeks	Yes	4–20	If used prior to pregnancy check diaphragm size at six weeks when involution is complete.
Condom/ Femidom	As soon as required	Yes	2–15	

*Persona is a system that predicts the fertile time in a woman's cycle. Persona monitors luteinising hormone and oestrone-3-glucuronide (a metabolite of oestradiol) through the use of urine test sticks.

**Lactational amenorrhoea is the use of breastfeeding to inhibit ovulation, therefore acting as a contraceptive. If a woman has a baby of less than six months, is fully breastfeeding and is ameorrhoeic there is only a 2% chance of pregnancy.

The earliest time of ovulation following a full-term delivery in non-breastfeeding women is around day 28. Therefore most hormonal methods are started at day 21.

Newcastle Postpartum Guidance Group 2005. Schering.

Chapter 8

Further supporting information

- Male and female reproductive system diagrams.
- The menstrual cyle.
- BMI chart.
- Combined oral contraceptive pill and emergency contraceptive pill international equivalents.
- Fraser Guidelines.

Male and female reproductive systems

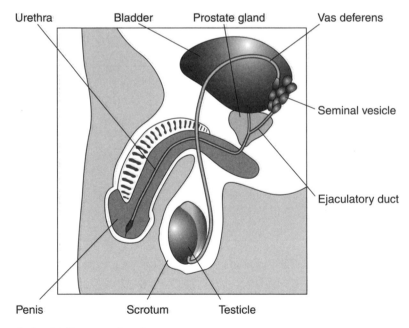

Figure 8.1 Male reproductive organs.

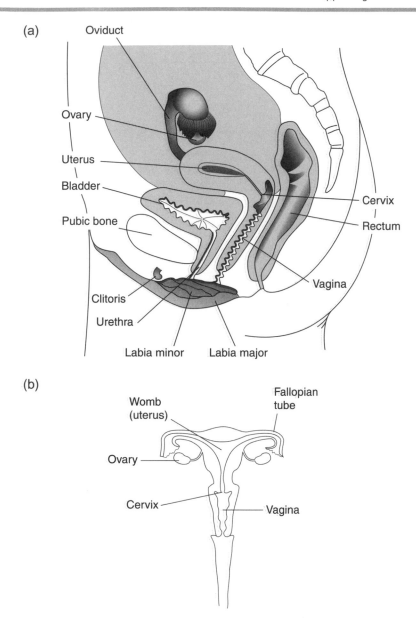

Figure 8.2 Female reproductive system.

The female reproductive system: physiological overview

Feedback control of ovarian hormone production

Box 8.1

- The pathway leading to the secretion of female steroid sex hormone begins in the hypothalamus, with secretion of the releasing hormone GnRH (gonadotrophin-releasing hormone).

- GnRH stimulates the pituitary to release FSH (follicle-stimulating hormone) and LH (luteinising hormone).
- FSH and LH stimulate the production of sex steroids oestradiol – the most common oestrogen (E2 in Figure 8.3) – and progesterone (P in Figure 8.3).
- Negative and positive feedback by oestradiol and progesterone controls FSH and LH production:
  - low levels of E2 and P cause negative feedback to inhibit FSH and LH secretion
  - high levels of E2 and P stimulate FSH and LH secretion.

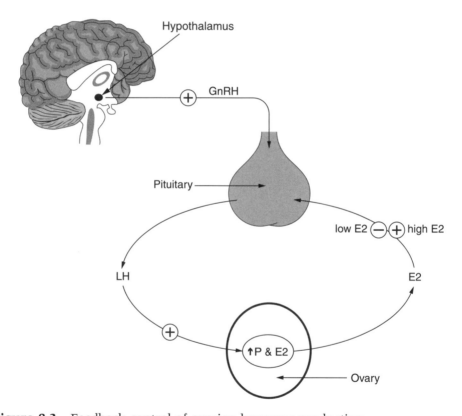

Figure 8.3 Feedback control of ovarian hormone production.

The menstrual cycle

Box 8.2

1 Follicular phase
   a The menstrual cycle begins as FSH stimulates development of an ovarian follicle. As this follicle matures, it begins producing a small but steady rising amount of oestradiol. This low level of oestradiol causes:
      i negative feedback: inhibition of FSH and LH secretion
      ii growth of the lining of the uterus.
2 Ovulation
   a The amount of oestradiol secreted at mid-cycle has increased to the high level that stimulates a surge of FSH and LH release by the pituitary.
   b The LH surge causes ovulation; the follicle ruptures and releases its egg near the opening of its fallopian tube.
3 Luteal phase
   a Following the release of its egg the follicle changes into a hormone-secreting structure, the corpus luteum, and secretes oestradiol and progesterone in response to LH:
      i oestradiol and progesterone stimulate the continued development of the lining of the uterus.
   b If pregnancy does not occur, the corpus luteum eventually disintegrates and stops secreting oestradiol and progesterone. The uterine lining sheds and menstruation occurs.
   c If pregnancy occurs the placenta produces hCG (human chorionic gonadotrophin) which maintains the corpus luteum's secretion of progesterone.
   d At three months' gestation the placenta takes over secretion of progesterone.

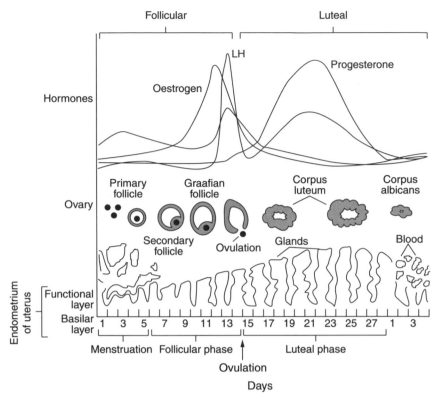

Figure 8.4 The menstrual cycle.

BMI chart

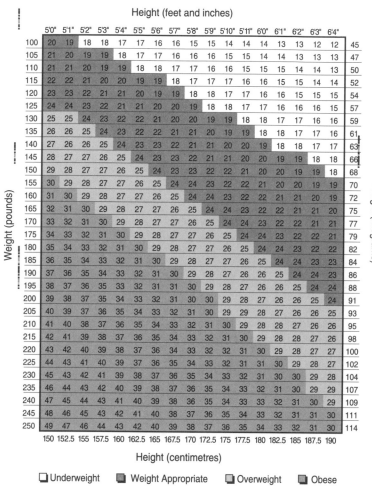

Figure 8.5   BMI chart.

International pill equivalents

Microgynon/Ovranette   30 mcg + 150 mcg levenorgestrel (LNG)

Ciclo, Ciclon, Combination 3, Contraceptive LD, Egogyn, Egogyn 30, Femigoa, Follimin, Gynatrol, Levelen, Levora, Lo-Femenal, Lo-Gentrol, Lo-Ovral, Lo-Rondal, Lorsax, Mala D, Microgest, Microgyn, Microvlar, Minibora, Minidril, Minigynon 30, Minivlar, Min-Ovral, Mithuri, Neo-Gentrol 150/30, Neomonovar, Noevletta, Nordet, Nordette 150/30, Nogestril Pill, Norgylene, Norvetal, Ologyn-Micro, Ovoplex 30/150, Ovoplexin, Ovral L, Ovranet, Riget, Rigevidon, Sexcon, Stediril 150/30, Stediril 30, Stediril M, Suginor.

Microgynon 20   20 mcg + LNG 100 mcg

Alesse, Balancelle, Loette, Leios, Micro-Levten, Miranova, Levlite.

Cilest   35 mcg + norgestimate 250 mcg
Effiprev, Effiprev 35, Ortho-Cyclen, Cyclen, Maclex, Neofam.

Femodene/Minulet   35 mcg + gestodene 75 mcg
Ciclomex, Evacin, Femodeen, Feminol, Femovan, Gestodene, Ginera, Ginoden, Gynera, Gynovin, Lerogin, Minulette, Moneva, Myvlar.

Femodette   20 mcg + gestodene 75 mcg
Harmonet, Meliane, Minigeste, Microgen, Minifem, Clclomex 20, Diminut, Melodene, Fedra, Femiane, Feminot 20.

Marvelon   30 mcg + desogestrel 150 mcg
Cycleane 30, Desogen, Desolette, Frilovon, Marviol, Microdiol, Novelon, OrthoCept, Pructil 21, Prevenon, Regulon, Varnoline, Lovina 30, Cicliclon, Desmin 30, Desoran, Gynostat 30.

Logynon/Trinordiol   Ethinyloestradiol (EE) 30 mcg + LNG 50 mcg
                     EE 40 mcg + LNG 75 mcg
                     EE 30 mcg + LNG 125 mcg
Fironetta, Levordiol, Modutrol, Triagynon, Triciclor, Triette 21, Trigoa 21, Trigynon, Trikvilar, Tri-Levlen, Trionetta, Triovlar, Triphasil, Triquilar, Triquilar ED, Tri Regal, Trisiston, Tri-Stediril, Triviclor, Trolit, Trivora, Trifas, Trifeme, Nova-step.

Ovysmen/Brevinor   35 mcg + norethisterone (NET) 500 mcg
Brevicon, Conceplamite, Genora, Gynex 0.5/35E, Intercon 5/35, Mikro Plan, Modacon, Modicon NEE 0.5/35, Nelova 0.5/35E, Neo-Ovopausine, Nilocan, Norminest, Orthonett-Novum, Ovacon, Ovysmen 0.5/35, Perle LD.

Loestrin 30   30 mcg + norethisterone acetate 1500 mcg
Loestrin 1.5/30, Logest 1.5/30, Minestril-30, Zorane 1.5/30, Econ Mite, Mala N, Trentovlane.

Loestrin 20   20 mcg + norethisterone acetate 1000 mcg
Loestrin 1/20, Lostrin 21 1/20, Minestril-20, Minestrin 1/20, Loestrin Fe 1/20.

Tri Novum   EE 35 mcg + NET 500 mcg
             EE 35 mcg + NET 750 mcg
             EE 35 mcg + NET 1000 mcg
Ortho 777, Ortho-novum 777, Triella.

Levonelle
Estinor, Madonna, Nerlevo, Plan B, Postinor 2, Rigesoft, Vikela.

Dianette
Diane 35, Brenda 35, Tina, Juliet 35ED.

Yasmin
Pettibelle.

Consent and the Fraser Guidelines

Young people under the age of 16 are legally able to consent to or refuse treatment provided the health professional has assessed their understanding of the procedure and any possible consequences. The Human Rights Act 1998[1] and the United Nations Convention on the Rights of the Child,[2] to which the UK is a signatory, state that the wishes of a young person must be taken into account when considering their best interests. The Children Act 1989 gave children the authority to consent to and refuse treatment.[3]

In England the legal age for heterosexual and homosexual intercourse is 16 years. However, although not legal, children between the ages of 13 and 15 are considered able to consent to sexual intercourse. Children below the age of 13 are deemed legally incompetent to consent to sexual activity and as such all sexual intercourse would be considered non-consensual.[4]

There was some confusion in the early 1980s regarding the issuing of contraceptives to girls under 16 and whether their parents should be involved. In 1974 the Department of Health and Social Security (DHSS) issued a memo of guidance to doctors advising that contraceptive advice could be given to girls aged under 16 without informing their parents but that they should always ask the girl's permission to tell her parents. However, the memo was followed up in 1980 by an adage: the need to persuade the girl to involve her parents or guardian and that this decision to involve the parents or not lay with the clinician. Naturally the way this was interpreted varied widely between clinicians. Some carried on as before, advising and issuing contraception to under 16s and encouraging the young woman to talk to her parents; other young people were told they would have to bring their parents to the appointment. As a result young people felt that confidential advice and treatment were not available to under 16s.

Eventually, following one mother's unsuccessful attempt to gain assurance that her daughters would not be provided with contraceptive advice or treatment without her consent, clearer and more explicit guidelines were produced. These guidelines made it clear that health professionals could provide contraceptive advice and treatment to young people provided that certain conditions were met. These conditions are called the Fraser Guidelines,[5] named after the judge who presided over the case. Each time a young person consults for treatment, an assessment should be made of their competence to consent.

This judgement referred specifically to doctors but it is considered to apply to other health professionals working with young people. It may also be interpreted as covering youth workers and health promotion workers who may be giving contraceptive advice and condoms to young people under 16, but this has not yet been tested in court.

Health professionals are able to provide contraceptive advice and treatment to under 16s as long as the following conditions are met:

- The young person understands the professional's advice.
- The young person is encouraged to inform their parents.
- The young person is likely to begin, or to continue having, sexual intercourse with or without contraceptive treatment.
- Unless the young person receives contraceptive treatment, their physical or mental health, or both, are likely to suffer.
- The young person's best interests require them to receive contraceptive advice or treatment with or without parental consent.

Although these criteria specifically refer to contraception, the principles are deemed to apply to other treatments, including abortion.

NB: Similar provision is made in Scotland by the Age of Legal Capacity (Scotland) Act 1991. In Northern Ireland, although separate legislation applies, the then Department of Health and Social Services Northern Ireland stated that there was no reason to suppose that the House of Lords' decision would not be followed by the Northern Ireland Courts.

References

1 Cabinet Office (1998) *Human Rights Act 1998*. HMSO, London.
2 United Nations General Assembly (1989) *United Nations Convention on the Rights of the Child*. United Nations, New York.
3 Cabinet Office (1989) *Children Act 1989*. HMSO, London.
4 Cabinet Office (2003) *Sexual Offences Act 2003*. HMSO, London.
5 *Gillick v West Norfolk and Wisbech Area Health Authority* (1985) 1 AC 12, 184 G.

Section 2

Sexual health

Chapter 9

Introduction to integrated sexual health services

What is sexual health?

The World Health Organization in 2002 defined sexual health as:

> a state of physical, emotional, mental and social wellbeing related to sexuality; it is not merely the absence of disease, dysfunction or infirmity. Sexual health requires a positive and respectful approach to sexuality and sexual relationships, as well as the possibility of having pleasurable and safe sexual experiences, free of coercion, discrimination and violence. For sexual health to be attained and maintained, the sexual rights of all persons must be respected, protected and fulfilled.[1]

Sexual health is now being recognised as something that not only impacts on each area of an individual's life, but also that each area of an individual's life impacts and influences the ability to maintain their sexual and reproductive health. Health needs to be encompassed under a holistic vision in order to optimise maintaining the health of our nation.

Sexual health may be compromised by problems associated with sexually transmitted infections (STIs) and human immuno-deficiency virus (HIV), unintended pregnancy or sexual dysfunction. A range of medical conditions, mental health problems and acute or chronic illness can also have an impact on sexual health.[2]

Consequences of poor sexual health can include:

- pelvic inflammatory disease, which can cause ectopic pregnancies and infertility
- HIV
- cervical and other genital cancers
- hepatitis, chronic liver disease and liver cancer
- recurrent genital herpes
- bacterial vaginosis and premature delivery
- unintended pregnancies and abortions
- psychological consequences of sexual coercion and abuse
- poor educational, social and economic opportunities for teenage mothers.[3]

With the move towards integrated service provision, sexual and reproductive health professionals have a duty to proactively help define, facilitate and support sexual and reproductive health and wellbeing in the community.

The poor sexual health of the nation is now widely acknowledged and reflected in substantial rises in rates of sexually transmitted infections (STIs), HIV and unwanted pregnancy. The UK,[2] Welsh,[4] and Scottish[5] national strategies for sexual health and HIV call for comprehensive services provided in a range of clinical settings responsive to patients' needs.

In order to facilitate the move towards integrated service provision within services, the healthcare professional will need to acquire the skills so that whatever scenario presents itself through the service doors, they will be able to deal with it, or have a pathway of referral to support the issues arising.

STI case management is the care of a person with an STI-related syndrome or with a positive test for one or more STIs. The components of case management include: history-taking, clinical examination, correct diagnosis, early and effective treatment, advice on sexual behaviour, promotion and/or provision of condoms, partner notification and treatment, case reporting and clinical follow-up as appropriate. Thus, effective case management consists not only of antimicrobial therapy to obtain cure and reduce infectivity, but also comprehensive consideration and care of the patient's reproductive health.[6]

In this section of the book, we will guide you through the practical and operational tools that have aided in our progress and service provision.

We have included:

- how to take a comprehensive sexual health history
- the physical examination
- testing
- diagnosis
- treatment.

Taking a sexual health history

Taking a sexual health history has consistently been seen as a taboo area by those who do not work in the field on a regular basis. Yet the principles of asking pertinent sexual health questions should not differ from the principles applied in any consultation. What one must be aware of is one's own embarrassment at asking the questions; this may in turn promote embarrassment with the client or patient and potentially lead to an unproductive consultation.

The keys to a good consultation are as follows:

- Consideration of your environment (if asking about sexual health, ensure sexual health literature/health promotion is seen visibly).
- The arrangement of the seating (respect physical space but do not isolate the client or patient).
- Confidentiality – this is of the utmost importance when exploring sexual health issues; it must be promoted right from the first contact with the reception, in the waiting environment and during a consultation. The service confidentiality statement should be made known to all staff and clients and discussed before any questions are asked. An example of a confidentiality statement from our service is given in the box.

Suggested statement:

'We are a confidential service. We will not tell anyone else that you have been here unless you give us permission to do so. We work as part of a team, so information that you give one member of staff may be shared with another. If you do not want this to happen then please tell us. However, if we are told any information that you or someone else is at serious risk of being hurt, for example being abused by someone, then we may have to tell someone else. But we would always talk it through with you first.'

- See the client on their own where possible, even under 16-year-olds. All clients have the right to confidentiality regardless of age.
- Introduce yourself and explain your role or designation. Check that the client's details are correct and ask if it is all right to use their first name.
- Explain to the client that you will be asking personal, maybe emotive or embarrassing, questions. It must be highlighted that these questions are asked of everyone and are used in order to determine the correct tests required as well as pathways of referral and treatment options.
- Decide whether to use colloquialism or medical language. When in consultation, it is important to recognise the population you serve, which can dictate the level of language you may use. As health professionals, terminology can become very medical based but it is not always necessary to use this level of language. Remember that clues can be gained from listening to the client and gauging what they come to you with, rather than you dictating the overall level of the consultation. Reflecting what the client says is also helpful in determining if there is a common understanding on both sides.
- The best way to get an explanation to a question is to ask open-ended questions. This may not always be appropriate but is useful when trying to get the client's perspective on the problem, issue or condition. Examples of open-ended questions are:
  - 'How can I help you today?'
  - 'How long have you had this difficulty?'
  - 'Do you have any other problems when having sex?'[7]

Proformas

Good history-taking and structured sexual health assessment by trained staff can help services to effectively and efficiently identify people's sexual health needs. Such a system may take the form of structured case-note sheets and proformas. Structured assessment and history-taking sheets can support consistent practice, provide appropriate documentation, facilitate audit and be used as a basis for developing integrated care pathways.[6]

Developing a proforma, or a sexual history-taking sheet, to use in practice can be very useful. Proformas are thought-provoking and standardise practice across a service. Some may argue that it takes away from the health professionals' ability to think for themselves. On the other hand, a proforma is directional in a consultation, can be applied to a time-limited consultation and is easily accessed for reference in a set of clinical/client notes.

An example of a clinic proforma for sexual health assessment is included (*see* Figure 9.1). The second proforma is a young person's assessment sheet (*see* Figure 9.2); this has been drawn up in consideration of issues pertaining to young people's sexual health and confidentiality issues.

| CHYPS AND WYPS SEXUAL HISTORY SHEET | Name/Clinic no: _____ Dob: _____ | City and Hackney **NHS** Teaching Primary Care Trust |

Client History Date: _____ **Seen By:** _____

CLIENT PLACE OF BIRTH: TIME RESIDENT IN U.K (IF APPLICABLE):

NO. OF SEXUAL PARTNERS IN LAST 3/12	1	2	3	4
Last sexual intercourse (SI)				
Sexual partner: Male/Female Regular / Casual or other Duration of relationship				
Protected or unprotected Vaginal/ anal / oral or other SI				
PARTNER: Country of origin: _____ STI diagnosis or symptoms				

PAST HISTORY OF STI inc HIV (Diagnosis/Treatment history/Contact tracing):

HISTORY OF COERCION: YES ☐   (SEE NOTES)   NO ☐

PAST MEDICAL/SURGICAL HISTORY INC: HISTORY OF BLOOD TRANSFUSION	MEDICATION

ALLERGIES: YES ☐   NO ☐   PENICILLIN ALLERGY: YES/NO /DON'T KNOW   DETAILS:

CIGARETTE SMOKER: YES ☐   NO ☐   AGE STARTED: ☐   AMOUNT PER DAY:

RECREATIONAL DRUG USE INC:IVDU OR PAST HX OF SEXUAL PARTNERS IVDU	ALCOHOL: YES ☐ NO ☐
	WHAT KIND:
	UNITS/WEEK:
	DISCUSS IF PERCIEVED PROBLEM

Figure 9.1   Clinic proforma – sexual health.

LMP: CYCLE: REG / IRREG: PCB: ☐   IMB: ☐

DATE:	PREGNANCIES	DELIVERY TYPE/ANY COMPLICATIONS:

LAST CX SMR: WHEN/WHERE   **RESULT:**

ABNORMAL SMEAR HISTORY:

HEPATITIS VACCINATION HISTORY:

CONTRACEPTION HISTORY/PREGNANCY RISK/TEST:

EXAMINATION: **LAST PU'D:**

INGUINAL NODES:

OTHER:

FOLLOW UP INFORMATION GIVEN AND CONTACT TRACING:

RETURN: WHEN   **or RESULTS LETTER: WHEN**   **SIGNATURE/DESIGNATION/DATE:**

CLINIC CARD GIVEN WHERE APPLICABLE:

FOLLOW UP INFO:

Figure 9.1   (*continued*)

CHYPS AND WYPS YOUNG PERSON'S PROFORMA	Name/Clinic no: _____ Dob: _____	City and Hackney **NHS** Teaching Primary Care Trust

EXPLANATION OF SERVICES AND PROVISIONS ☐

EXPLANATION OF CONFIDENTIALITY ☐

REASON FOR ATTENDANCE:

FRASER COMPETENCY IF UNDER 16 YEARS OLD:

PARENTAL CONSENT AND INVOLVEMENT HAS BEEN EXPLORED WITH THE YOUNG PERSON	
THE YOUNG PERSON WILL CONTINUE TO HAVE UPSI WITH OR WITHOUT TREATMENT	
THERE IS RISK TO THE YOUNG PERSON'S PHYSICAL/MENTAL WELL BEING IF ADVICE OR TREATMENT WITHELD	
IT IS IN YOUNG PERSON'S BEST INTEREST TO GIVE ADVICE OR TREATMENT	
AGE OF CURRENT PARTNER	

DETAIL OF PARENTAL RESPONSIBILITY, NATURE OF SEXUAL RELATIONSHIPS AND ANY REPORTED HISTORY OF COERCION

Figure 9.2 Young person's proforma.

ALCOHOL USE: Yes / No

Type/ Amount / frequency:

DRUG-USE:

TYPE	Y OR N	AMOUNT	FREQUENCY
CIGARETTES			
CANNABIS			
ECSTASY			
CRACK			
COCAINE			
HEROIN			
SPEED			
SOLVENTS			
LSD			
OTHER			

Related risk taking behaviour:

DISCUSSED IF CLIENT PERCIEVES A PROBLEM WITH DRUGS / ALCOHOL: Yes / No

REFERRAL TO DRUGS / ALCOHOL AGENCY OFFERED? Yes / No   Accepted / Declined

If accepted, referred to whom:

PREGNANCY TEST: YES [   ]   NO [   ]   RESULT [   ]

CONDOM DEMONSTRATION GIVEN: YES [   ]   NO [   ]

[   ]

CONDOMS GIVEN: YES [   ]   NO [   ]   HOW MANY

ANY FURTHER ACTION:

COMPLETED BY:SIGNATURE/DESIGNATION: Date:

Figure 9.2   (*continued*)

Sexual history flowchart

The following flowchart pertains to what is required for comprehensive sexual history-taking. This can be adapted to local need, consultation time and service setting. Explanatory notes are included to assist in supporting why the questions are being asked.

History of complaint

Male

- Discharge, colour, consistency, dysuria, frequency in urination or lower back pain
- Testicular or other unusual pains
- Bowel habit change
- Lumps, lesions +/− pruritis
- When symptoms began and duration
- Recent travel abroad
- When last passed urine

Female

- Discharge, colour, consistency/discomfort, dysuria, itching, frequency in urination
- Lower abdominal or lower back pain
- Bowel habit change
- Dyspareunia – deep pain during sex
- Lumps, lesions
- When symptoms began and duration
- Recent travel abroad

Number of sexual contacts in last three months

- When, who – regular/casual, duration of relationship, if contactable
- Protected or unprotected sex – receptive or active oral/vaginal/anal or other
- Contacts with country of origin, if recently travelled or sex abroad
- Contacts symptomatic?

History of STIs and cervical smear history

- What STI, when and where diagnosed and treated and if followed up
- History of vaccination for hepatitis A or B, when and if completed schedule
- When last cervical smear taken, where and result
- Any abnormal smears or treatment history

Coercion

- Any history of coercive sex?
- Assess Fraser competency in under 16-year-olds
- *See* Figure 9.2

Questions:
- Do you enjoy having sex?
- Are you happy in your relationship?
- Have you ever felt forced into having sex when you did not want to? How did you deal with this? How did this leave you feeling?

Medical history

- Present or past illness, relevant family medical history
- Allergies (especially to antibiotics or other medications)
- Medication at present or antibiotics in last three weeks
- Any problems with sexual performance or desire

Social history

- Alcohol intake, recreational drug use including smoking, intravenous drug user (IVDU) or sex with IVDU
- History of blood transfusions, piercings or tattoos
- Explore family if applicable – children, home, job
- Review for under 16s according to Fraser guidance
- *See also* Figure 9.2

Menstrual history

- LMP (last menstrual period)
- Normal or irregular bleed
- Usual cycle pattern
- Intermenstrual bleeding or postcoital bleeding history

Obstetric history

- Number of pregnancies, parity/terminations/miscarriages/ectopic pregnancies
- Any complications?
- Breastfeeding presently?

Contraceptive history

If condom use, usual type preferred
Any accidents or problems reported
Condom demonstration offered
Type of contraception used, duration and compliance
Pregnancy risk assessment

Sexual history-taking questions – explanatory notes

	Explanatory notes
History of complaint	This should come from the client's or patient's perspective where possible, with clarification around whether or not symptoms not mentioned may also be present, looking at the following:
	• When did the symptoms begin (during sex, after sex, in a non-sexual activity)?
	• Where is the discharge or pain coming from (throat, vagina, penis or anus, skin)?
	• Frequency – do the symptoms occur all the time or 'on and off'?
	• Has the client taken any medication for the symptom or used any other remedial therapies?
	• Have these worked or been effective in any way?
	• Have they had this symptom or problem before? What happened at the time if they have?
	• Is this problem precipitated or worsened by any factor (movement, urination, sex)?
Number of sexual contacts in last 3 months	• Are the sexual contacts male or female? What is the client's perceived sexual orientation?
	• Ascertain whether or not any sexual partner(s) has any signs or symptoms of infection or has been diagnosed with infection.
	• Is it too early to test for infection (i.e. less than seven days post-sexual intercourse)?
	• Consider window period of three months for HIV, syphilis and testing for hepatitis infection.
	• Was the sex abroad or with someone who has recently travelled from abroad? (Consider resistant infection, hepatitis B and HIV risks.)
	• Number of partners where unprotected sex occurred? This can help determine whether or not there needs to be risk reduction discussion and risk assessment in terms of acquiring an infection and risk of pregnancy.
History of STIs and cervical smear history	• Again this will determine risk reduction discussion and risk assessment in acquiring infection, ongoing complication of infection (PID/subfertility) and risk of pregnancy.

Explanatory notes

- How recent or distant was the infection diagnosed or treated?
- Was the sexual partner(s) at the time tested and/or treated?
- Cervical smear history – relevant for visual observation in clinical examination, and also to monitor uptake in accordance with the national cervical screening programme.

Coercion: sexual abuse, sexual assault, sexual violence, grooming

- This may prove a difficult question to ask but should be explored where possible.
- It is important to acknowledge that we all have different interpretations of what coercive sex may mean, and if this is disclosed the client's perspective on what they call coercion should be explored before being acted upon.
- Pathways of referral or support should be put in place before embarking on asking this question, for if a 'Pandora's box' is opened, the issues need to be dealt with and referred effectively.

Considerations are:

- sexual assault guidelines or referral pathways
- young people's guidelines and child protection policy
- counselling/psychology support services
- referral to interagency professionals such as the health adviser.

Medical history

- Medical conditions: diabetes, heart disease, blood pathologies – sickle cell), osteoarthritis.
- Blood transfusion – in the UK or abroad?
- Have there been any gynaecological operations or interventions?
- Are there any medications being taken that may affect testing or treatment options?
- Are there any medications being taken that can affect sexual performance (antidepressants, antipsychotics, heart medication, herbal remedies, anti-epileptics)?

Social history

- Alcohol and recreational drug use is asked both as a health promotion exercise and also to ascertain risk-taking behaviour and vulnerability in a public arena (e.g. if goes out alone and binge drinks or takes drugs in non-familiar environments/with strangers).
- IVDU or sex with IVDU, history of blood transfusion pre-screening or in third world country, piercings or tattoos with unclean or non-sterilised equipment – risk of HIV/hepatitis B or C transmission.

	Explanatory notes
	• Explore family life to see the whole picture of the client complaint or reason for attendance. Also this gives the opportunity to see if any further support needs are required, e.g. referral to social services or other agency. • In under 16s it is important to explore who has parental responsibility, the client's living arrangements, school/college attendance and ages of sexual contact(s). *See* Fraser Guidelines.
Menstrual history	• Irregular or intermenstrual bleeding may be indicative of an STI/ectopic pregnancy/miscarriage.
Obstetric history	• Parity will support what is seen on observation during clinical examination. • If risk of existing pregnancy, other pregnancy history will support reaching a diagnosis in any symptoms expressed (lower abdominal pain, dyspareunia) or health education needed.
Contraceptive history	• Is there a pregnancy risk due to unprotected sex? • Are there any issues with current contraception – discuss. • Is a condom/Femidom demonstration needed? • Is client aware of emergency contraception information and local access? • Are there any contraindications to current medication being taken or to be prescribed? • If Implanon *in situ* – observe site, when inserted? • If IUS or IUD *in situ* – observe for threads on examination, when inserted and any issues arising.

References

1 World Health Organization (2002) *International WHO Technical Consultation on Sexual Health*. 28–31 January. WHO, Geneva.
2 Medical Foundation and Sexual Health (medFASH) (2005) www.medfash.org.uk/publications/documents/Recommended_standards_for_sexual_health_services.pdf
3 Department of Health (2001) *Sexual Health and HIV Strategy*. HMSO, London.
4 Welsh Assembly Government (2000) *Strategic Framework for Promoting Sexual Health in Wales*. National Assembly of Wales. www.cmo.wales.gov.uk/content/work/sexualhealth/sexual-health-strate.pdf
5 Scottish Executive (2000) *Enhancing Sexual Wellbeing in Scotland: a sexual health and relationship strategy*. Scottish Executive. www.scotland.gov.uk/sexualhealthstrategy/
6 Peck SA (2001) The importance of the sexual health history in the primary care setting. *Journal of Obstetric, Gynaecological and Neonatal Nursing*. **30**: 269–74.
7 Camden PCT (2004) *Eliciting a Sexual History. A video training pack for healthcare professionals*. Camden PCT.

Chapter 10

Clinical examination

Clinical examination

The physical examination allows healthcare professionals to confirm the symptoms described by the client and check for signs of sexually transmitted infections (STIs). It is important to remember and respect that a client may refuse to be examined, even after counselling regarding what will happen and why it is important. It is therefore important to be aware of alternative ways of determining a diagnosis without a full clinical examination; however, it needs to be explained to the client that diagnosis without examination may be presumptive. This is also relevant where onsite microscopy (as a tool to determine preliminary diagnosis where applicable) is not available.

Examination of the vulva and perineum

1 Inspect the following structures:
    a Mons pubis – observe pubic hair for pubic lice, molluscum or other presentation.
    b Labia majora/minora – observe for inflammation, ulceration, swelling or nodules.

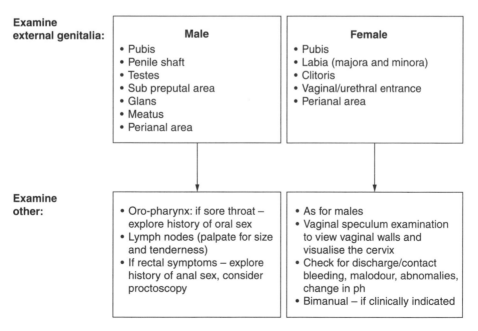

Examine external genitalia:

Male
- Pubis
- Penile shaft
- Testes
- Sub preputal area
- Glans
- Meatus
- Perianal area

Female
- Pubis
- Labia (majora and minora)
- Clitoris
- Vaginal/urethral entrance
- Perianal area

Examine other:

- Oro-pharynx: if sore throat – explore history of oral sex
- Lymph nodes (palpate for size and tenderness)
- If rectal symptoms – explore history of anal sex, consider proctoscopy

- As for males
- Vaginal speculum examination to view vaginal walls and visualise the cervix
- Check for discharge/contact bleeding, malodour, abnormalities, change in ph
- Bimanual – if clinically indicated

Figure 10.1 Clinical examination.

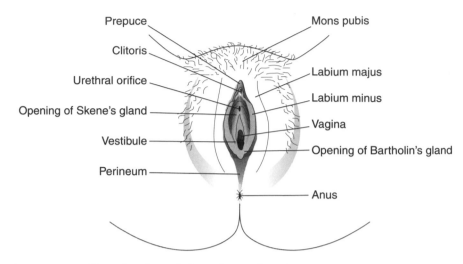

Figure 10.2 Examination of the vulva and perineum.

   c   Clitoris – observe for masculinisation (>2 cm).
   d   Urethral orifice – observe for discharge or prolapse.
   e   Vaginal opening or introitus – observe for inflammation, ulcerations, nodules, previous episiotomy scar, hymenal status.
   f   Perineum – observe for ulceration, nodules, genital warts or other presentation.
   g   Anus – observe for inflammation, discharge, ulceration, nodules, genital warts or other presentation.
   h   Observe for signs of female genital mutilation (FGM).
2 Palpate the following structures:
   a   Inguinal area – appreciate abnormal lymphadenopathy.
   b   Labia majora – appreciate Bartholin gland (pea size).

How to insert a speculum

- Warm with water or apply lubricating jelly (it is advised not to use lubricant if carrying out a cervical smear as it can obscure cervical cells on the slide).
- Touch inner thigh with speculum and ask patient if it is too warm or too cold.
- Ask patient to spread knees laterally to relax perineal musculature.
- Press fingers on perineal body and assess relaxation.
- Make sure speculum blades are closed and thumbscrew loosened.
- Gently insert index finger and assess location of cervix (anterior vs posterior). Not all practitioners perform this but it can be useful in locating the hard to reach cervix. You may be guided by any comment pertaining to previous difficulty from the patient's history.
- Insert speculum gently at 45-degree angle (pointing towards sacrum), avoid pinching vulva/introitus, avoid sensitive urethra and anterior vaginal wall.
- Gently open speculum and attempt to visualise cervix; if not visualised, assess speculum location if necessary, close speculum and insert more posteriorly (cervix will usually 'pop' into view).

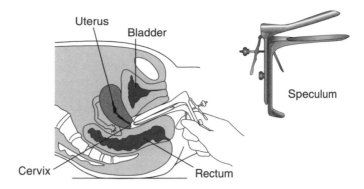

Figure 10.3 How to insert a speculum.

- Once cervix visualised, open blades more and stabilise cervix by tightening thumbscrew.
- Inspect the cervix:
  - observe position, prolapse, location of transformation zone, type of cervical os (multiparous vs nulliparous), ulcers, colour, polyps, plaques, contact bleeding, abnormal discharge, or bleeding from cervical os, cysts and nodules
  - abnormal findings include: ectropion, Nabothian cysts, pelvic inflammatory disease (purulent discharge), cervicitis, herpetic cervicitis, cervical polyp, previous obstetric lacerations, cervical carcinoma, cervical prolapse, spontaneous miscarriage.

Bimanual examination checklist

Bimanual examination	Palpate and record
Vagina	Cysts or masses
Cervix	
Consistency	Soft and/or firm
Mobility	Mobile or immobile
Tenderness	Tender or non-tender
Supra pubic	Masses or tenderness
Posterior cul de sac	Masses or tenderness
Uterus	
Size	Small or weeks gestation
Shape	Smooth or irregular
Position	Anteverted/flexed, retroverted/flexed, mid
Consistency	Soft or firm
Mobility	Mobile or immobile
Tenderness	Tender or non-tender
Adnexa	
Tubes/ovaries, ligament	Enlargement, masses or tenderness

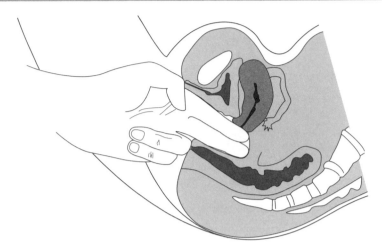

Figure 10.4 Bimanual examination.

Knowledge base required:

- anatomy of uterus and adnexa
- diseases affecting uterus and adnexa
- pathology of lesions of uterus and adnexa.

Male examination

Observation

- In general, the left testis lies a bit lower in the scrotum than the right. The testes should appear as two discrete swellings, although if the room is particularly cold, they may retract up towards the inguinal canal.
- First examine the glans (i.e. the head) of the penis.
- If the client is uncircumcised, draw back the foreskin so that you can look at the glans in its entirety. Make sure that you return the foreskin to its normal position at the end of the exam. Whether you withdraw the foreskin or you ask the patient to is discretionary.
- Look at the opening of the urethra. Make note of whether it is more or less at the tip of the penis, on the top side (known as epispadias) or on the bottom side (hypospadias).
- Observe along the shaft of the penis for skin presentations. Any obvious skin abnormalities on the penis, scrotum or surrounding areas?
- Examine at the base of the penis/amid the pubic hair for any skin abnormalities (e.g. pigmented areas, ulcers, vesicles etc.). You will obviously look more closely if the patient complains of seeing/feeling something in that region.
- Gently feel the testes, palpating the tissue between the thumb and next two fingers of your examining hand. Each should be of the same consistency and size.
- Explore with the client the issue and importance of testicular self-examination. Back up with literature where applicable.
- Make careful note of any discrete lumps or bumps within the body of the testis.

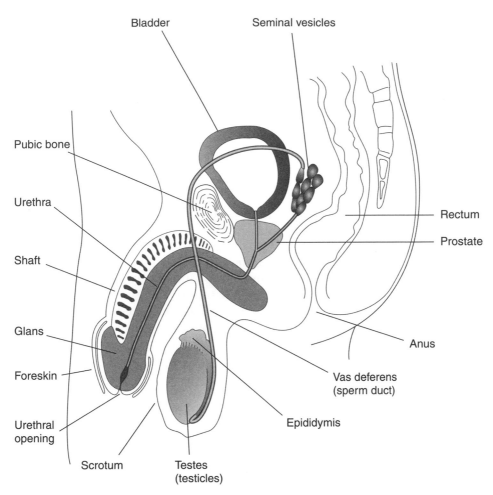

Figure 10.5 Male reproductive organs.

Chapter 11

Symptom flowcharts and testing guidelines

The following chapter gives guidance on how to take tests from the particular oro-genital sites for microscopy, where applicable, and/or culture. It has been made as generic as possible to facilitate practice across the board and thus in some areas may mean that the specific testing mediums or kits used in your service will have to be ascertained first. For the latest national guidance on testing in STIs, visit the British Association for Sexual Health and HIV website: www.bashh.org.

The guidance has been taken from the nursing guidelines as developed for our clinical service. These were developed for our service having been adapted and updated from the nursing guidelines (2000), given with kind permission by Jane Bruton, Clinical Nurse Lead, from the John Hunter Clinic, St Stephen's Centre, London.

The basic considerations and tools needed to perform the relevant tests are outlined in each section. In order for a clinical examination to take place examination rooms should ideally have:

- an examination chair or couch
- an appropriate light source for examination
- a curtain to maintain confidentiality – mobile or fixed.
- a client gown or cover sheet.

Considerations

Discharge/discomfort

Male

Consider:

- Non-gonococcal urethritis
- Chlamydia
- Gonorrhoea
- Genital ulceration
- Trichomonas
- UTI or non-specific infection
- Trauma or urethral obstruction

Female

Consider:

- Bacterial vaginosis
- Candida
- Trichomonas
- Chlamydia
- Gonorrhoea
- Retained foreign body
- UTI or non-specific infection

Lumps, spots or lesions

Consider:

- Genital warts
- Molluscum
- Abscess
- Folliculitis
- Skin tag
- Lice/scabies
- Haemorrhoids
- Dermatoses
- Balanitis (male)/Candida

Rectal discomfort

Consider:

- Gonorrhoea
- Chlamydia
- Herpes
- Syphilis
- Lympho granuloma venereum
- Chemical/physical trauma
- Genital warts, haemorrhoids
- Anal fissure/sinus
- Non-specific proctitis

Ulceration

Consider:

- Herpes
- Syphilis

- Bacterial infection
- Chemical or physical trauma
- Chancroid
- Lympho granuloma venereum

Abnormal vaginal bleeding

Consider:

- STI
- Cervical ectropian
- Neoplasm, polyp, endometrial pathology
- Fibroid
- Pregnancy
- Physical/chemical trauma
- Hormonal contraceptive changes

Female genital pain

Consider:

- Vaginal infection
- Ulceration
- Trauma
- Pelvic inflammatory disease
- Ectopic pregnancy
- Fibroids
- Ovulation/menstrual pain
- Referred bowel pain or haemorrhoids
- UTI

Routine tests

Test	Male	Female
Where microscopy is being performed	• Urethral smear for non-gonococcal or non-specific urethritis (NGU/NSU)/gonorrhoea	• Sample from lateral vaginal walls for candida and bacterial vaginosis • From posterior fornix for trichomonas
High vaginal swab	• N/A	• Sample from lateral vaginal walls for candida and bacterial vaginosis • From posterior fornix for trichomonas According to local policy, may only be performed in symptomatic patients
Gonorrhoea culture	• Urethra, throat, and rectum as applicable	• As with males • In addition endo-cervix
Chlamydia	• Urethra	• As with males • In addition endo-cervix
Bloods	• Syphilis treponemal serology • Hepatitis A, B, C as clinically indicated • HIV	• As with males
Urinalysis	• Check first-pass urine for clarity and threads if symptomatic • Perform urinalysis • +/– MSU (midstream urine) if clinically indicated	• Perform urinalysis • +/– MSU if clinically indicated • Pregnancy test if clinically indicated
Cervical cytology	• N/A	• Perform cytology as per national/local cytology guidelines • Perform cytology if clinically indicated
Viral swab	• From presenting lesions for herpes simplex virus (HSV) – type 1 or type 2	• As with males
Microscopy, culture and sensitivity (MC&S)	• Where bacterial or fungal infection suspected at a presenting lesion or site of infection	• As with males

Obtaining a throat swab for gonorrhoea

Equipment

- Non-sterile latex gloves.
- Tongue depressor.
- One charcoal transport medium with swab.

Action	Rationale
• Ask the client to sit with his/her head bent slightly backwards, facing a strong light source. Ask the patient to open his/her mouth wide.	• To ensure maximum visibility of the throat.
• Depress the tongue slightly with the tongue depressor, and then quickly, but gently, rub the swab over the faucial area or any area with a lesion or visible exudate.	• To obtain the required sample.
• Place the sample into the charcoal medium.	• To prepare for culture.

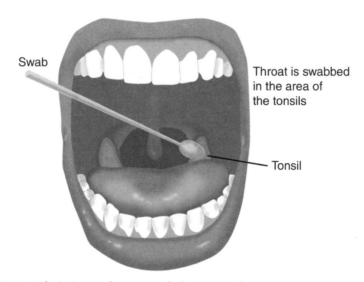

Figure 11.1 Obaining a throat swab for gonorrhoea.

Obtaining vaginal, cervical and urethral specimens

Please note: The testing procedure is clean, not aseptic.

Equipment

- Non-sterile latex gloves.
- Cuscoe speculum (metal or plastic) – size can be somewhat determined from obstetric history, the size of the client/client age.
- pH paper.
- Lubricating jelly (refer to local guidance on use of lubrication in examination and testing).
- Two cotton-tipped swabs – one for high vaginal and one for cervical gonorrhoea testing.

- One cervical chlamydia swab.
- Two fine cotton-tipped swabs – for gonorrhoea and chlamydia testing from the urethra.
- One bottle of chlamydia-testing medium, gonorrhoea-testing medium and testing medium for high vaginal tests.

Where microscopy is being performed:

- Cardboard tray.
- Two plain microscopy slides.
- One cover slip.
- Normal saline solution.

(*See also* section on 'Gram staining'.)

Action	Rationale
• Assist the client into the lithotomy position. Wipe away any secretions from the vulval area using a downward movement from the clitoris to the perineum.	• To enable inspection of the genital area and remove any excess secretion.
• Prior to inserting the speculum, sample discharge directly onto the pH paper.	• To assess acidity or alkalinity of the vagina.
• Warm the speculum to body temperature under a running tap for metal cuscoe *or* apply small amount of lubricating jelly to the speculum upper end and under side.	• To promote the comfort of the client. • To allow for the easy transition of the speculum into the vagina.
• Insert the speculum gently into the vaginal orifice. When fully inserted, open the speculum and locate the cervix. When the cervix is visualised and fixed at the mouth of the speculum, tighten the screw on the speculum to fix it into position.	• To ensure maximum visibility of the area to be inspected and swabbed.

Vaginal slides and swabs

Action	Rationale
Where microscopy is being performed: • Take two slides – leave one dry, and apply one drop of normal saline to make the other one wet.	

- Using one cotton-tipped swab, swab the lateral vaginal walls and spread the specimen evenly onto the dry glass slide, at the end furthest away from frosted end.
- Using the same swab, swab the posterior fornix; then dip it into the saline solution on the wet slide, and apply the cover slip.
- Go to posterior fornix for second time with new or same swab and place into high vaginal-testing medium.
- *Where microscopy is not being performed, omit the parts where specimen is placed on a glass slide. Take swabs and place directly in testing medium.*

- To obtain specimens from the vagina and prepare them ready for microscopy and culture.

- To test for candida and clue cells indicative of bacterial vaginosis.

- To test for trichomonas vaginalis.

Cervical slides and swabs

Action
- Gently clean the cervix using the cervix mop.
- Insert a cotton-tipped swab into cervical os, and rotate it 360°.
- *Where microscopy is being performed*: spread some of the sample obtained onto the dry glass slide, in the middle, and place swab in gonorrhoea-testing medium.
- Microscopy is not performed for chlamydia testing locally. The swab is taken from the endocervical area and placed directly into testing medium.
- For chlamydia test – refer to specific tesing kit guidance for how to take an appropriate sample.

- *Where microscopy is not being performed, omit the parts where specimen is placed on a glass slide. Take swabs and place directly in testing medium.*

Rationale
- To ensure maximum visibility of the cervix os.
- To obtain an adequate specimen for testing.
- To prepare the specimen for microscopy and culture.

- To obtain an optimum amount of endocervical cells for chlamydia culture. Different testing kits will carry specific instruction.

Urethral specimen

Action	*Rationale*
• Insert fine cotton-tipped plastic swab into the urethra for 1 cm in an upward and backward direction, and rotate the swab very gently.	• To obtain the required specimen.
• Spread the specimen evenly onto the dry microscopy slide, at the frosted end of slide, and then place into the gonorrhoea-testing medium.	• To prepare the specimen for microscopy and culture.
• Repeat insertion with the second fine cotton-tipped swab. For chlamydia test – refer to testing kit guidance for how to take an appropriate sample.	• To obtain an optimum amount of urethral cells for chlamydia testing.
• *Where microscopy is not being performed, omit the parts where specimen is placed on a glass slide. Take swabs and place directly in testing medium.*	

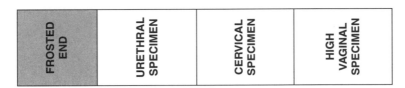

| FROSTED END | URETHRAL SPECIMEN | CERVICAL SPECIMEN | HIGH VAGINAL SPECIMEN |

Figure 11.2   An example of glass slide and specimen collection in women.

Obtaining urethral specimens (male)

Equipment

- Non-sterile gloves.
- One microscopy slide – where microscopy is being performed.
- Two fine cotton-tipped or plastic swabs.
- Cardboard tray.
- One chlamydia-testing medium.
- One gonorrhoea-testing medium.

Action	Rationale
• If the client has not been circumcised, ask him to retract the foreskin.	• To expose the urethra.
• Ask the client to gently part the meatus.	• To ensure maximum visibility of the area to be swabbed.
• Insert a fine cotton-tipped swab into the meatus, approximately 1.5–2 cm deep, and rotate it gently.	• To obtain the appropriate amount of sample.
• Where microscopy being performed, spread some of the sample obtained thinly onto a dry glass slide, then place the swab into the gonorrhoea-testing medium.	• To obtain the required specimen and prepare it for microscopy and culture.
• Repeat insertion with the second fine cotton-tipped swab. For chlamydia test – refer to specific testing kit guidance for how to take an appropriate sample.	• To obtain an optimum amount of urethral cells for chlamydia testing.
• *Where microscopy is not being performed, omit the parts where specimen is placed on a glass slide. Take swabs and place directly in testing medium.*	

Obtaining a subpreputial specimen

Equipment

- Non-sterile gloves.
- One microscopy slide – where microscopy is being performed.
- Cardboard tray.
- One cotton-tipped swab.
- One testing medium for MC&S.

Action	Rationale
• If the client has not been circumcised, ask him to retract the foreskin.	• To ensure maximum visibility of the area to be sampled.
• Gently swab the affected area.	• To obtain the required specimen.
• Where microscopy is being performed, spread some of the sample obtained thinly onto the dry glass slide. Then place swab into charcoal transport medium.	• To prepare the specimen for microscopy to look for evidence of candida, and to prepare for culture.
• *Where microscopy is not being performed, omit the parts where specimen is placed on a glass slide. Take swabs and place directly in testing medium.*	

Obtaining a urine sample for chlamydia testing

Equipment

- Clear plastic/glass receptacle.
- Urine-processing pouches (if used, as some laboratories require the specimen of urine only).

Sample collection and testing procedure may vary according to local guidance.

Action	Rationale
• Label container with client's details.	• To ensure correct identification of client's specimen.
• For women, ask client to wipe outside of vagina from front to back.	• To decrease the occurrence of possible inhibitory organisms.
• Ask client to pass minimum 15–20 ml of first-void urine into container. Allow urine to cool down for five minutes.	• To obtain sample for testing.
• Check expiry date of urine-processing pouches. Place one pouch into container with sample.	• To ensure sample is sent for testing correctly prepared.
• Secure container tightly.	• To prevent leaking specimens and compromise of infection control.

- Send off sample in a pre-labelled virology form.

- Store in refrigerator until transported to laboratory.

- Ensure it is ready for transportation, testing and reporting.
- To maintain viability of the sample.

Obtaining a slide and swab using a proctoscope

Equipment

- Non-sterile latex gloves.
- Lubricating jelly.
- Disposable proctoscope.
- Light source.
- One microscopy slide – where microscopy is being performed.
- Cardboard tray.
- One cotton-tipped or plastic swab.
- One gonorrhoea-testing medium.
- Tissues.

Refer to local guidance if first time or symptomatic proctoscopy examination.

Action	Rationale
• Assist the client into the left lateral position and ask him/her to draw his knees up to his/her abdomen.	• To ensure maximum visibility of the area to be examined and to ensure maximum safety for the client during the procedure.
• Lubricate the proctoscope and insert into the anus, and ask the client to bear down. When the proctoscope is fully inserted, remove the introducer and attach/use the light source (if available).	• In order to relax the anal sphincter and be able to examine the appearance of the rectal mucosa.
• Using a clean swab, swab the rectum with care. Then withdraw the swab and remove the proctoscope gently, inspecting the rectal mucosa as you do so.	• To obtain the required sample and to visualise the rectal mucosa.
• Where microscopy is being performed, spread the sample obtained onto a glass slide and then place swab in gonorrhoea-testing medium.	• To prepare the specimens for testing.

- Wipe away any excess lubricant around the anus.
- *Where microscopy is not being performed, omit the parts where specimen is placed on a glass slide. Take swabs and place directly in testing medium.*

- To make the client comfortable.

Note

If a rectal specimen is required for chlamydia testing, the chlamydia culture transport medium *must be used* straight from the refrigerator.

Summary of NHS cervical screening programme

The NHS cervical screening programme has recently issued new guidelines for cervical screening nationally, implemented in April 2005.

The cervical screening programme now invites women from age 25, and routine screening ends at age 65.

This has been changed because the incidence of cervical cancer under 25 years is very low. One in six smears taken under 25 is abnormal with high prevalence of low-grade lesion. In 2002, there were 55 000 abnormal smears, 26 cases registered as cervical cancer and there were five deaths from this disease among the age group of 20–24.

The frequency of screening has also been revised (*see* table).

Age	Frequency of screening
< 25	First invitation
25–49	Three yearly
50–64	Five yearly
65 +	Only screen those who have not been screened since age 50 or those who have had recent abnormal tests

Referral guidelines for colposcopy

Type of abnormal smear test	Number of tests	Recommended for referra	Colposcopy appointment waiting times
Inadequate smear	Three consecutive tests	90%	Within eight weeks
Borderline squamous cells nuclear changes	Three consecutive tests	90%	Within eight weeks
Abnormal tests of any grade	Three abnormal tests in ten years	90%	Within eight weeks
Borderline nuclear changes of endocervical cells	One test	100%	Within two weeks
Mild dyskaryosis	One test	90%	Within eight weeks
Moderate dyskaryosis	One test	90%	Within four weeks
Severe dyskaryosis*	One test	90%	Within four weeks
Possible invasion	One test	100%	Urgent referral (90% seen within two weeks)
Glandular neoplasia	One test	100%	Urgent referral (90% seen within two weeks)
Abnormal cervix	Suspicion of cancer	Urgent referral	Urgent referral (90% seen within two weeks)
Women with symptoms	IMB/PCB over 40 (under 20 sexual health screen first)	Urgent referral	Urgent referral (90% seen within two weeks)
Previous treatment for CIN	One test	100%	Urgent referral (90% seen within two weeks)

*Dyskaryosis: cervical screening uses cytology to detect areas of nuclear abnormalities, which are described as dyskaryotic.
CIN: cervical intra-epithelial neoplasia; IMB: intermenstrual bleeding; PCB: postcoital bleeding.

The smear result may come back with additional infections indicated, such as the following:

Actinomyces-like organisms (ALOs)

ALOs on smear results require no specific intervention in the vast majority of patients. They are usually seen in patient using an IUD or IUS.

If the patient is asymptomatic:

- The IUD does not need to be removed, nor is there need for antibiotics.
- The patient should be informed.
- The patient should be given an appointment to discuss the findings.
- There is a small chance of developing pelvic actinomycosis; therefore the client should have six-monthly follow-up to assess symptoms by pelvic and abdominal examination.
- If the patient wishes to remove the device there is no need to send it for culture.

If the patient is symptomatic (symptoms include pelvic pain, deep dyspareunia, intermenstrual bleeding, vaginal discharge, dysuria, pelvic tenderness):

- The device should be removed and sent for culture. A course of antibiotics should be given (penicillin/amoxicillin/erythromycin).

Bacterial vaginosis

If bacterial vaginosis is reported, treatment is not required unless the patient is symptomatic or pregnant.

Candidiasis

Treatment is not required unless symptomatic.

Herpes simplex

All patients should be screened for STIs or referred to a sexual health clinic for screening and treated if infection is active.

Trichomonas vaginalis

Treatment is required. All patients should be screened for STIs or referred to a sexual health clinic for screening. The cervical screening sample may not be satisfactory due to marked inflammatory changes. Repeat cervical cytology screening after treatment.

Pregnant women

If a woman has been called for routine screening and she is pregnant, the test should be deferred. If the previous test was abnormal the test should not be delayed but should be taken in the second trimester unless there is a clinical contraindication. A routine cervical smear should be taken three months following the delivery.

Post-hysterectomy (total)

All women in the cervical screeing age range undergoing a hysterectomy and who have had a negative screening test do not need a vault smear. Women with a subtotal hysterectomy should continue with the routine screening programme.

Immunosuppressed women

Women who are on immunosuppression therapy should have routine screening according to their age.

HIV-positive women

These women should have yearly cervical screening tests. The age range is the same.

Obtaining a cervical smear

Practice statement

To screen a woman for precancerous changes in the cervix by obtaining cells from the squamo-columnar junction.

Equipment

- Cuscoe vaginal speculae.
- Non-sterile gloves.
- Aylesbury spatula.
- Lubricating jelly.
- Box for transporting slides.
- Request forms.
- Cytology fixative.
- Tissues.
- Cytobrush.
- One frosted-end slide.

Action	*Rationale*
• Check client and GP's address. Obtain consent to send result to GP and home address. Document in client notes.	• To ensure confidentiality is maintained and to ensure client understands, and remains/ becomes part of the national cervical recall system.
• Check the client is not menstruating.	• Unable to get adequate sample during menstruation.
• Assist client into lithotomy position. Select appropriate type of speculum.	• To ensure comfort for the client.
• Warm speculum to body temperature under running tap (metal cuscoe). Apply a very thin layer of lubricating jelly to speculum.	• To ensure comfort for the client and allow for the easy transition of the speculum into the vagina.

- Pass the speculum gently. When it is fully inserted open the speculum to visualise the cervix and tighten the screw on the speculum to fix it in position.
- Observe the cervix, noting the clinical appearance.

- Insert the spatula into the cervical os using the bilobed end. Firmly rotate the spatula 360° – two turns.
- Spread the material thinly (but not too scantily) onto the glass slide using gentle longitudinal strokes.
- A cytobrush may be used in conjunction with the spatula (check local policy). Insert gently into the os and rotate 360°.
- If both brush and spatula are used, one sample will be put on one half of the slide and one on the other half.
- Flood the slide with cytology fixative *immediately* and leave to dry.

- Remove the speculum gently and offer tissues.
- Ensure clear labelling of slides (in pencil) to correspond with the request form. Give references to past cytology.

- So that an accurate smear can be obtained and obvious abnormalities detailed on the request form.

- To ensure that the smear spans the squamo-columnar junction at all points.
- To obtain a single cell layer on as much of the slide as possible without damaging the cells.

- So that an accurate smear can be obtained.

- To ensure each specimen is easily identified.

- To give a well-preserved specimen and to ensure immediate, adequate fixation of cells as air-drying disrupts the cell structure.
- To fix cervical sample ready for transportation and testing.
- To ensure client comfort.

- To ensure correct identification of sample with client.

NB: *If a smear is done as part of a sexual health screen and infection is confirmed, the smear should be discarded. Equally if marked cervicitis or inflammatory changes are observed, then the smear should be deferred.*

Please also note that the introduction of liquid-based cytology (LBC) in the very near future will mean that the above prescribed way of taking a cervical smear will ultimately become obsolete. LBC uses a brush technique which places the sample in a medium which is processed in the lab in a way that ensures even distribution of cells on the slide.

Obtaining a specimen for viral culture

Equipment

- Non-sterile latex gloves.
- Viral culture transport medium.
- One swab.

Action	Rationale
• Firmly swab the lesion, rotating the swab and taking care not to touch the surrounding skin. Place the swab directly into the transport medium.	• To obtain an uncontaminated specimen for culture.
• Label each swab with site of specimen.	
• Be aware if samples need to be virus typed.	• If taken for herpes simplex virus, to ascertain if type 1 or 2.
• Store the specimen in the refrigerator until it is sent to the laboratory.	• To prolong virus survival.

Obtaining a blood sample

Equipment

- One pair of close-fitting gloves.
- Tourniquet.
- Sterile alcohol wipe (refer to local guidance on use of this in venepuncture).
- Cotton wool balls.
- Sterile elastoplast or hypoallergenic tape.
- Appropriately sized needle for venepuncture system (most commonly 21 gauge in adults).
- Appropriately sized and type of syringe for test required.
- Specimen forms and transport bags.

The procedure

- Identify the patient and ensure you have the correct patient records.
- Explain the procedure and allow the patient time for questions and, if desired, withdrawal of consent.
- Ask the patient whether or not he or she has had blood taken previously. He or she may be aware of particular problems encountered and of the best site available.
- Spend time selecting the most appropriate vein in order to achieve successful venepuncture at the first attempt. This promotes patient confidence and is more comfortable.

- Wash your hands.
- Attach needle to syringe. If more than one sample is required, and using a plunger-type syringe, create a vacuum in the other syringes.
- Apply tourniquet to upper arm and rotate limb to face you. Palpate and examine arm to distinguish between veins, tendons and arteries. The vein should be firm and bouncy. Clenching and unclenching the patient's fist can help, but may lead to a minor alteration in test results.
- Put on gloves and clean area with alcohol swab, allowing to dry passively for 30 seconds.
- Stretch the skin over the vein with thumb of one hand. Insert the needle, bevel side up, into the vessel at a 30–45 degree angle. Do this smoothly: unnecessary swiftness can lead to puncture of the vessel wall; being too slow increases discomfort.
- Stabilise the needle and syringe with your thumb, index finger and middle finger of one hand and withdraw the syringe's plunger with the other. If blood flows, click the plunger into locked position; otherwise, if using vacutainer, allow the blood to flow to required quantity.
- If further samples are required, unlock the syringe while stabilising the needle with the other hand, then connect the next syringe.
- Once all the samples have been collected, release the tourniquet and cover the needle with cotton wool, but do not apply pressure until you have withdrawn the needle, as this causes unnecessary pain and venous damage.
- Apply firm pressure for 30–60 seconds to prevent bruising. Check the site. If clotted apply elastoplast or gauze and tape.
- After completing the procedure, dispose of the needle and syringe and any contaminated waste in the appropriate container.

Points to remember

- If the tourniquet has been on for more than two minutes prior to inserting the needle, release and allow blood to return to the hand before reapplying.
- If a venous valve is entered during the procedure, the patient will feel sudden, acute pain. Discontinue the procedure immediately.
- If after two attempts you are unsuccessful, seek assistance from a colleague.
- Observe the patient throughout the procedure for signs of dizziness, fainting or paraesthesia.
- Be aware that the brachial artery is also sited near the sites most commonly used for venepuncture.

This section has closely referred to 'Venepuncture: a quick reference guide'. *Nursing Standard* (1999) **13**: 36.

Microscopy and Gram staining

The Gram-staining process is a laboratory staining technique that distinguishes between two groups of bacteria by the identification of differences in the structure of their cell walls. The Gram stain, named after its developer, Danish bacteriologist Christian Gram, has become an important tool in bacterial taxonomy, distinguishing between so-called Gram-positive bacteria, which remain coloured after the staining procedure, and Gram-negative bacteria, which do not retain dye. The staining technique can be seen in the following table.

Following solvent treatment, only Gram-positive cells remain stained, possibly because of their thick cell wall, which is not permeable to solvent. After the staining procedure, cells are treated with a counterstain, e.g. a red acidic dye such as safranin or acid fuchsin, in order to make Gram-negative (decolourised) cells visible. Counterstained Gram-negative cells appear red, and Gram-positive cells remain blue. Although the cell walls of Gram-negative and Gram-positive bacteria are similar in chemical composition, the cell wall of Gram-negative bacteria has a thin layer between an outer lipid-containing cell envelope and the inner cell membrane. This means that within the staining process, the cell wall loses the crystal violet colour during the use of the alcohol in the decolourisation process and takes on the red stain at the end part of the staining process. The Gram-positive cell wall is much thicker, and retains the crystal violet stain even through the decolourisation process.

Gram staining

Practice statement

To prepare and stain the slides correctly for oil immersion microscopy.

Equipment

- Non-sterile gloves.
- Hot plate.
- Running water.
- Laboratory coat or apron.
- Slide tray.
- Staining rack.
- Blotting paper.
- *Staining bottles containing:*
  - crystal violet (the primary stain)
  - iodine solution (the mordant by forming a crystal violet–iodine complex)
  - decolouriser (ethanol is a good choice)
  - safranin (the counterstain)
  - water (preferably in a squirt bottle or from a specified tap).

Action	Rationale
- Dry the slide thoroughly on the hot plate.	- To fix the specimen onto the slide.
- Place the slide on the staining rack. Apply methyl violet or crystal violet. Leave for one minute.	- Stains all the organisms and the background purple.

- Wash off the methyl violet with water. Apply Lugol's iodine and leave it on for one minute.
- Iodine fixes the methyl violet into the Gram-positive organisms.
- Wash off iodine with acetone until no more colour comes away (approximately 2–3 seconds). Put the slide under running water immediately.
- Acetone decolourises all methyl violet from the background and Gram-negative organisms. Water stops the decolourisation process.
- Apply safranin as a counterstain. Leave for one minute.
- Stains the background and Gram-negative organisms red.
- Wash the safranin off with water.
- To remove excess stain.
- Remove excess water with blotting paper and dry slide on the hot plate.
- The slide needs to be dry ready for oil immersion microscopy.

Microscopy diagnosis tool

High vaginal swab dry prep to look for:
- lactobacilli
- candida (hyphae and spores)
- mixed vaginal flora, at varying gradients
- clue cells (alongside clinical signs, used in the diagnosis of bacterial vaginosis)
- at 100× magnification – high-powered field.

High vaginal wet prep to look for:
- trichomonas
- candida spores and hyphae under fluorescent illumination
- at 40× or 60× magnification – low-powered field.

Cervix and urethral dry prep to look for:
- polymorphonucleocytes
- polymorphonucleocytes containing diplococci Gram-negative pairs (intracellular only – indicative of gonorrhoea)
- at 100× magnification – high-powered field.

Chapter 12

Infections and treatment guidelines

The following sections contain descriptions of each sexually transmitted infection (STI). For each infection the following areas are examined:

- the nature of the infection
- aetiology
- prevalence
- incubation period
- symptoms
- possible findings
- diagnosis
- treatment
- follow-up advice.

The treatment guidelines have been adapted from the guidelines from our clinical service. They were written with guidance from the local departments of sexual health, microbiology department and using national guidance from the British Association for Sexual Health and HIV (BASHH) and the British National Formulary (BNF) (March 2005).

Only the most commonly used treatment options have been listed for simplicity sake but further information can be gained with reference to the above resources.

These are meant as a guide only and you should refer to local guidance on microbial resistance and locally agreed treatment options (pharmacy department) before you develop your own service treatment guidelines.

Kc60 codes

Below is a list of diagnosis codes known as Kc60 codes. Each infection has a code attributed to it and they are used in contact tracing or partner notification, as well as a way of contributing to the national picture of prevalence of infection.

The Communicable Diseases Surveillance Centre, otherwise known as the Health Protection Agency (HPA), compiles data on genitourinary (GU) clinics' cases of STIs and monitors infection rates.

More information and data (Kc60 codes) are available by the number of cases of specific STIs seen at genitourinary medicine (GUM) clinics, NHS trusts and, in some cases, individual hospital clinics through the Health Protection Agency (HPA) website: www.hpa.org.uk.

Your contribution

As a service we made a decision that we wanted our data reflected in the national system. We had traditionally provided data through our local department of sexual health but have now made arrangements to provide data independently.

As a service, it is important to think about how you will contribute to national statistics as by doing so it will help to give a truer reflection of the national profile of infection and provide a source from which you can audit your local prevalence data.

A summary of rare and tropical infections, e.g. chancroid and donovanosis, has been included for the reader's information. However, their diagnosis, treatment and management should be carried out by level three centres and informed by local microbiology departments.

Similarly the sections on hepatitis, syphilis and HIV and AIDS focus on pre-test discussion aspects of the infection, as once a diagnosis is made treatment is co-ordinated by specialist centres; in addition treatment regimes are complicated and rapidly evolve.

Kc60 codes

A1	Primary syphilis
A2	Secondary syphilis
A3	Early latent syphilis
A4	Cardiovascular syphilis
A5	Central nervous system
A6	Late latent syphilis
A7	Congenital syphilis <2 years
A8	Congenital syphilis >2 years
B1	Uncomplicated gonorrhoea
B2	Prepubertal gonorrhoea
B3	Gonococcal ophthalmia neonatorum
B4	Epidemiological treatment of suspected gonorrhoea
B5	Complicated gonococcal infection including: PID/epididymitis
C1	Chancroid
C2	Donovanosis
C3	LGV (lymphogranuloma venereum)
C4A	Postpubertal uncomplicated chlamydia
C4B	Complicated chlamydia infection including: PID/epididymitis
C4C	Uncomplicated chlamydia infection
C4D	Chlamydia ophthalmia neonatorum
C4E	Epidemiological treatment of suspected chlamydia
C4H	Uncomplicated non-gonococcal/non-specific infection in males/RX of mucopurulent cervicitis in females
C4I	Epidemiological treatment of NGU
C5	Complicated infection (non-chlamydial/non-gonoccoccal) including: PID/epididymitis

C6A   Trichomonas
C6B   Anaerobic/bacterial vaginosis and anaerobic balanitis
C6C   Other vaginosis/vaginitis/balanitis
C7A   Anogenital candidiasis
C7B   Epidemiological treatment of C6 and C7
C8   Scabies
C9   Pediculosis pubis
C10A   Anogenital herpes simplex – first attack
C10B   Anogenital herpes simplex – recurrence
C11A   Anogenital warts – first attack
C11B   Anogenital warts – recurrence
C11C   Anogenital warts – re-registered cases
C12   Molluscum contagiosum
C13A   Antigen-positive viral hepatitis B – first diagnosis
C13B   Numbers of first diagnosis which were acute viral hepatitis B
C13C   Viral hepatitis B – subsequent presentation
C14   Viral hepatitis C – first diagnosis

D2A   Urinary tract infection
D2B   Other conditions requiring treatment at GUM
D3   Other episodes not requiring treatment

E1A   Asymptomatic HIV infection – new diagnosis
E1B   Asymptomatic HIV infection – subsequent presentation (not AIDS)
E2A   Symptomatic HIV infection – new diagnosis (not AIDS)
E2B   Symptomatic HIV infection – subsequent presentation (not AIDS)
E3A   AIDS – first presentation – new HIV diagnosis
E3A2   AIDS – first presentation – HIV diagnosed previously
E3B   AIDS – subsequent presentation

P1A   HIV antibody test – no GU screen
P1B   HIV antibody test – offered and refused
P2   Hepatitis B vaccination – first dose only
P3   Contraception – excluding: condom provision
P4A   Cervical cytology – minor abnormality
P4B   Cervical cytology – major abnormality

S1   Sexual health screen – no HIV antibody test
S2   Sexual health screen with HIV antibody test

Definition of organisms

Bacteria

Responsible for gonorrhoea, including gonococcal pelvic inflammatory disease (PID), syphilis.

Mycoplasmas and chlamydiae

These are bacteria but they do not have rigid cell walls; mycoplasmas can be responsible for non-gonoccocal urethritis (including chlamydial) and cervicitis. Chlamydia trachomatis is primarily responsible for chlamydial PID.

Viruses

The smallest known disease-causing agents, viral STIs, include hepatitis B and C, genital herpes, molluscum contagiosum, human papilloma virus (HPV – genital warts), and the human immunodeficiency virus/acquired immune deficiency syndrome (HIV/AIDS).

Fungi

Plant-like organisms causing candidiasis.

Protozoa

Single-celled microscopic forms of animal life – responsible for trichomoniasis.

Metazoa

All other parasitic animal life forms, i.e. scabies and pediculosis.

Bacterial vaginosis (BV)

Background

Bacterial vaginosis (BV) is the commonest cause of abnormal discharge in women of childbearing age. It is characterised by an overgrowth of predominantly anaerobic organisms (*Gardnerella vaginalis*, *Prevotella* species, *Mycoplasma hominis*, *Mobiluncus species*) in the vagina, leading to replacement of lactobacilli and an increase in pH from as low as 4.5 to as high as 7.0. It can arise and remit spontaneously in sexually active and non-sexually active women. It is more common in black women than white, those with an intrauterine contraceptive device, and those who smoke. It is not regarded as a sexually transmitted infection. The aetiology is not known.

BV and PID

The incidence of BV is high in women with pelvic inflammatory disease (PID); however, there are no prospective studies investigating whether treating asymptomatic women for BV reduces their risk of developing PID subsequently.

BV and pregnancy

- BV is common in some populations of women undergoing elective termination of pregnancy (TOP), and is associated with post-TOP endometritis and PID.
- In pregnancy BV is associated with late miscarriage, preterm birth, premature rupture of membranes, and postpartum endometritis.

Symptoms

- Offensive vaginal discharge ('stale fish').
- Worse after coitus or menses.
- Approximately 50% asymptomatic.

Signs

- Not associated with soreness, itching or irritation.
- Offensive odour, moderate white/grey–white homogeneous discharge.

Diagnosis

- Discharge as above.
- pH >4.5.
- Malodour.
- Amine test positive (release of a fishy odour on adding alkali [10% KOH] to discharge).
- Gram stain for clue cells.

Treatment

BV

Drug	Formulation	Dosage	Frequency	Duration
Metronidazole	Oral tablets	400–500 mg OR 2 g	bd Stat	5–7 days

Allergy

Allergy to metronidazole is uncommon. Use 2% clindamycin cream for allergic women.

TOP/pregnancy/breastfeeding

- Reduction in post-TOP infection when BV treated with oral metronidazole or clindamycin cream before termination.
- In pregnant women treatment is indicated and the antenatal caregiver should be informed.

- Metronidazole enters breast milk and may affect its taste. The manufacturers recommend avoiding high doses if breastfeeding. Small amounts of clindamycin enter breast milk. It is prudent therefore to use an intravaginal treatment for lactating women.

Follow-up

Test of cure (TOC) is unnecessary if symptoms resolve.

Management

- Avoidance of vaginal douching, use of shower gel and use of antiseptic agents or shampoo in the bath.
- Asymptomatic non-pregnant women may not need treatment.
- Recurrences are common.

Sexual partners

Routine screening and treatment of male and female partners is not indicated.

Recurrences

For recurrent symptomatic BV, one option is suppressive therapy. The use of metronidazole gel 0.75% twice weekly for four to six months to decrease symptoms, after an initial treatment daily for ten days, is being evaluated. An alternative strategy is to use metronidazole orally 400 mg bd for three days at the start and end of menstruation, combined with fluconazole 150 mg as a single dose if there is a history of candidiasis also.

Balanitis

Background

Balanitis is a common condition, defined as inflammation of the glans penis, often involving the prepuce (balanoposthitis). It is a collection of disparate conditions with similar clinical presentation and varying aetiologies.

Possible causes:
- *Candida albicans*
- trichomonas
- streptococci group A and B
- anaerobes
- *Gardnerella vaginalis*
- *Staphylococcus aureus*
- *Mycobacteris*
- syphilis
- herpes simpex virus (HSV)

- HPV
- skin disorders such as: psoriasis, lichen sclerosus
- miscellaneous – trauma, irritants, poor hygiene, allergy.

Symptoms

- Local rash, soreness, itching, odour.
- Discharge from the glans/behind foreskin.
- Inability to retract foreskin.
- Associated symptoms: rash elsewhere on body, joint pains, swollen/painful glands.

Signs

- Ulceration.
- Scaling.
- Fissuring exudates.
- Crusting.
- Sclerosis.
- Oedema.
- Erythema.

Diagnosis

- Subpreputial swab for candida and bacterial culture.
- If ulceration present – herpes simplex culture and dark ground for spirochaetes.
- Syphilis serology.
- Culture for trichomonas if female partner has undiagnosed discharge.
- Screening for other STIs – particularly screening for chlamydia trachomatis infection/non-specific urethritis if a circinate-type balanitis is present.

Treatment (as for candida)

Candida

Drug	Formulation	Dosage	Frequency	Duration
Clotrimazole*	Cream 1%	20 g	bd	Until symptoms settle
Miconazole** Nystatin	Cream 2% Cream	As above 100 000 units/g	bd	If resistance suspected or allergy to imidazoles

* Effect on latex condoms and diaphragms not known.
** Product damages latex condoms and diaphragms.

- Fluconazole 150 mg stat orally if symptoms severe.
- In cases where inflammation is present the alternative use of Canesten hydrocortisone/Daktocort creams are useful.

Anaerobic infection

Symptoms

- Foul-smelling discharge.
- Swelling.
- Inflamed glands.

Signs

- Preputial oedema.
- Superficial erosions.
- Inguinal adenitis.
- Milder forms also occur.
- Subpreputial culture (to exclude other causes).

Treatment

- Metronidazole 400 mg twice daily for one week.
- The optimum dosage schedule for treatment is unknown.

Alternative regimen

- Co-amoxiclav 375 mg three times daily for one week.
- Clindamycin cream applied twice daily until resolved.
- These treatments have not been assessed in clinical trials.

General advice

- Saline bathing with weak solution twice daily while symptoms persist.
- Avoid soaps while inflammation present.
- Advise effect on condoms if creams supplied.
- Patients should be given a detailed explanation of their condition with particular emphasis on the long-term implications for their health (and that of their partner where a sexually transmissible agent is found).
- GU screen for other STIs – especially chlamydia and NSU.

Follow-up

Not necessary unless symptoms are severe and an underlying problem is suspected.

Management

Balanitis is a clinical diagnosis and covers a range of heterogenous conditions. The recommendations for management are therefore given on an individual basis.

Sexual partners

High rate of candidal infection in sexual partners. Sexual partners should be offered screening.

Candidiasis ('thrush')

Background

'Thrush' is a yeast-like fungus that is commonly carried as a commensal. It is present in the vagina of about one in five women with no symptoms. Causative agents include, most commonly, *Candida albicans* and non-albicans species. The clinical symptoms caused by albicans and non-albicans species are indistinguishable.

Symptoms

- Non-offensive vaginal discharge may be curdy.
- Irritation and/or soreness.
- Superficial dyspareunia.
- External dysuria.

Signs

- Erythema.
- Oedema.
- Fissuring.
- Satellite lesions.

Diagnosis

- pH 4–4.5 (pH >5 – suspected bacterial vaginosis or trichomonas vaginalis).
- Gram stain for pseudohyphae spores (may detect 65–68% of symptomatic cases).
- Culture – useful to confirm diagnosis in recurrent cases.

Treatment

Candida

Drug	Formulation	Dosage	Frequency	Duration
Clotrimazole*	Pessary	500 mg	Stat	
Clotrimazole*	Pessary	200 mg	Once at night	3 nights
Clotrimazole*	Vaginal cream (1%)	20 g	Twice daily	5–7 days

*Effect on latex condoms and diaphragms not known.

Pregnancy or breastfeeding

Oral therapy contraindicated. Treat with topical azoles – consider longer courses.

Follow-up

TOC is unnecessary unless symptomatic.

Management

- Asymptomatic non-pregnant patients may not need treatment.
- Avoid local irritants and tight-fitting synthetic clothing.

Sexual partners

Treatment is unnecessary if asymptomatic.

Recurrences

- Four or more episodes of symptomatic candidiasis annually: refer.
- Poorly understood.
- Exclude diabetes mellitus.
- Association with recent cunnilingus.
- Other risk factors include underlying immunodeficiency, corticosteroid use, frequent antibiotic use.

Chancroid

Background

Haemophilus ducreyi, the microbial agent of chancroid, used to be the most common cause of genital ulcers in many parts of the world. The pattern of genital ulcer disease (GUD) is changing, however, and recent studies have found that while GUD attributable to herpes simplex virus type 2 (HSV-2) infection is increasing, *H ducreyi* is decreasing in many areas.

H ducreyi is also known to be an important cofactor in the transmission of HIV infection, its diagnosis and treatment, assuming therefore even greater importance. Chancroid has been a rare occurrence in industrialised countries.

Co-infections of chancroid with *Treponema pallidum* or herpes simplex virus (HSV) are frequent.

The incubation period ranges between three and ten days. There are no prodromal symptoms.

The ulcer is classically described as:

- single or (often) multiple
- not indurated ('soft sore')
- with a necrotic base and purulent exudate
- bordered by ragged undermined edges
- bleeding easily on contact.

For diagnosis, treatment and management advice refer to your local microbiology department, hospital of tropical medicine, department of sexual health or www.bashh.org.

Chlamydia

Background

Chlamydia genital infection is an intracellular organism caused by the bacterium *Chlamydia trachomatis*. The chlamydia opportunistic screening pilot studies, involving women under 25, in Portsmouth and the Wirral have found higher prevalences of chlamydia (approximately 10%) than previously reported in selected populations.[1] Currently the chlamydial prevalence in men as well as women in the general population is unknown. Infection in the community is sustained by unrecognised and thus untreated symptomless infection both in men and women. Approximately 40% of non-gonococcal urethritis is caused by *C trachomatis*.[2]

Quality of specimens

- The sample must contain cellular material. Swabs should be inserted inside the cervical os and firmly rotated against the endocervix.
- Inadequate specimens reduce the sensitivity of all diagnostic tests.
- Urethral swab in men should be inserted 1–4 cm and rotated once before removal.
- There is no consensus on how to take a urethral swab in women.

Chlamydia (Females: uncomplicated)

Incubation

The incubation period is 14–21 days.

Symptoms

- Asymptomatic in up to 80%.
- Vaginal discharge.
- Menstrual disturbances, intermenstrual bleeding, postcoital bleeding.
- Lower abdominal pain/dyspareunia.
- Urethral syndrome.
- Anal – asymptomatic or discharge/discomfort.
- Pharyngeal – usually asymptomatic.

Signs

- Often normal appearance.
- Cervicitis.
- Occasional mucopurulent cervical discharge.
- Proctitis.

- Pelvic tenderness.
- Cervical excitation.

Diagnosis

- Nucleic acid amplification techniques (NAAT) taken from the cervix and urethra (10–20% additional positives will be detected by assaying a urethral specimen as well).
- If patient declines urethral or cervical swabs, first-void urine can be taken (20 ml).
- Chlamydia culture may be taken in selected cases (e.g. sexual assault) from relevant sites, e.g. pharynx/rectum.

Treatment

Chlamydia

Drug	Formulation	Dosage	Frequency	Duration
Doxycycline	Oral tablets	100 mg	bd	7 days
Azithromycin	Oral tablets	1 g	Stat	Use in pregnancy or breastfeeding only when there is no other alternative available.

Pregnancy or breastfeeding

Drug	Formulation	Dosage	Frequency	Duration
Erythromycin	Oral tablets	500 mg	qds	7 days
Erythromycin	Oral tablets	500 mg	bd	14 days
Amoxicillin	Oral tablets	500 mg	tds	7 days

Follow-up

At seven days, to check compliance, sexual abstinence and partner notification. Patients do not need to be retested for *C trachomatis* after completing treatment with doxycycline or azithromycin unless symptoms persist or re-infection is suspected. A TOC should be considered three weeks after the end of treatment with erythromycin. A TOC earlier will miss late failures and may detect non-viable organisms.

Management

- Offer full GU screen.
- No sex until therapy completed and partner(s) tested/treated.
- Issue contact slips to client to give to relevant sexual partner(s) in last six months.

Sexual partners

- Examine for STIs.
- Offer epidemiological treatment.

Complications

- Bartholin's abcess.
- Perihepatitis.
- Pelvic inflammatory disease (PID).
- Sexually acquired reactive arthritis (SARA).
- Adult conjunctivitis.

Treatment

Refer as appropriate.

Chlamydia (Males: uncomplicated)

Incubation

The incubation period is 14–21 days.

Symptoms

- Asymptomatic in up to 50%.
- Urethral discharge.
- Dysuria.
- Anal – asymptomatic or discharge/discomfort.

Signs

- Often normal appearance.
- Urethral discharge.
- Meatitis.
- Proctitis.

NB:
- Urine to have been held for at least one hour before being tested.
- Chlamydial infection may be present in the absence of urethritis.

Diagnosis

- Nucleic acid amplification techniques (NAAT) taken from the urethra.
- If patient declines urethral swabs, first-void urine can be taken (20 ml).
- NAAT not recommended for use for pharynx/rectum chlamydia testing.
- Chlamydia culture may be taken in selected cases (e.g. sexual assault) from relevant sites, e.g. pharynx/rectum.

Treatment

See Chlamydia (Females).

Follow-up

See Chlamydia (Females).

Management

See Chlamydia (Females).

Sexual partners

See Chlamydia (Females).

Complications

- Epididimo-orchitis.
- Sexually acquired reactive arthritis (SARA).
- Adult conjunctivitis.

Treatment

Refer as appropriate.

Donovanosis

Background

Donovanosis is a STI that usually manifests itself as genital ulceration. It is seen chiefly in small endemic foci in tropical countries. The causative organism, formerly *Calymmatobacterium granulomatis*, has recently been officially redesignated *Klebsiella granulomatis*.

Clinical features at site of primary inoculation

- One or more papules/nodules developing into friable ulcers or hypertrophic lesions which gradually increase in size. Lesions tend not to be painful.
- Regional lymph nodes: initially swelling of the nodes, followed (particularly in case of inguinal nodes) by spread of infection into overlying tissues, resulting in either abscess formation (pseudobubo) or ulceration of the overlying skin.
- Untreated infections may either resolve spontaneously or persist and slowly spread. Primary lesions of mouth and cervix occur and the latter have often been mistaken for malignant lesions.

- Complications include haemorrhage, genital lymphoedema, genital mutilation and cicatrisation, development of squamous carcinoma and, on rare occasions, haematogenous dissemination to bone and viscera (particularly during pregnancy).

For diagnosis, treatment and management advice refer to your local microbiology department, hospital of tropical medicine or department of sexual health.
Also refer to: www.bashh.org.uk.

Genital warts (anogenital)

Background

Anogenital warts are caused by the human papilloma virus (HPV), of which over 90 genotypes have been identified. The mode of transmission is most often by sexual contact but may be transmitted perinatally and from digital lesions. Most anogenital warts are benign and caused by types 6 and 11. Some lesions may contain oncogenic types associated with genital tract dysplasia and cancers. Anogenital warts are the 'tip of the iceberg' of genital infection with HPV as many people without warts have subclinical disease or latent infection.

Symptoms

- The large majority of genital warts result in little physical discomfort; however, they can be disfiguring and psychologically distressing.
- They may cause irritation and soreness, especially around the anus.
- Symptoms of distortion of urine flow or bleeding from the urethra, or anus, may indicate internal lesions.

Signs

- Perianal lesions are common in both sexes, but are seen more commonly in homosexual men.
- Warts in the anal canal are associated with penetrative anal sex, and may indicate the need for samples to be taken from the ano-rectal region for other STIs, e.g. *N gonorrhoeae* or *C trachomatis*.
- Occult lesions may be seen on the vagina, cervix, urethral meatus and anal canal. Extragenital lesions may be seen on the oral cavity, larynx, conjunctivae and nasal cavity.

Clinical appearances of exophytic warts

- Warts may be single or multiple.
- Those on the warm, moist, non-hair-bearing skin tend to be soft and non-keratinised and those on the dry hairy skin firm and keratinised.
- Lesions may be broad based or pedunculated and some are pigmented.

Diagnosis

- Clinical (biopsy/colposcopy).
- Examine the external anogenital and surrounding skin under good illumination.
- Females: vaginal speculum.
- Both sexes: proctoscopy may be indicated if history of anal receptive sex, or following clearance of perianal warts. Meatoscopy and proctoscopy should be performed if there is a history of distortion of urine flow or bleeding from the urethra or anus. Occasionally urethroscopy is indicated for more proximal warts.
- Classify warts as to morphology.
- Recording of lesions on genital maps at each visit is useful, providing a visual record of approximate number, distribution and response to treatment.
- Extragenital sites (e.g. oral cavity) examined if clinically indicated.

Treatment

- All treatments have significant failure and relapse rates.
- Treatment decisions should be made after discussing the appropriate options with the patient, taking into account their preference and convenience.

HPV/anogenital warts – soft

Drug	Formulation	Dosage	Frequency	Duration
Warticon Podophyllotoxin	Paint	–	bd for 3 days then 4 days without	Maximum 4-week course
Podophyllin	15–20% solution	–	1× or 2× week in clinic and washed off 4 hours later	
Trichloroacetic acid (TCA)			1× week in clinic	

HPV/anogenital warts – keratinised

Cryotherapy
Excision
Electrocautery

Imiquimod (any wart type)	5% cream		3× week, washed off 6–10 hours later	16 weeks

- Treatment may involve discomfort and local skin reactions. Written information on management of treatment side effects is recommended.
- Local anaesthetic creams plus or minus injection with e.g. lignocaine 2% could be used before ablative therapy to minimise discomfort. Adrenaline-containing anaesthetic should be avoided for lesions on the penis and around the clitoris.
- 5-FU: this is a DNA antimetabolite cream. Teratogenic and severe side effects, no longer recommended.
- Interferon: cream or injection, expensive and systemic side effect, but may give low relapse rate as adjunct to laser treatment. Consultant advice required.

The immunosuppressed respond poorly with increased relapse rates and dysplasia.

Suggested treatment according to anatomical sites

- *Urethral* – standard treatment if base of lesion visible (if not, refer to urologist); caution as treatment may cause adhesions or stenosis.
- *Intra-anal* – TCA/cryotherapy/electrocautery. Treatment of uncertain benefit in asymptomatic.
- *Perianal* – consider general surgery referral.
- *Vaginal* – TCA/cryotherapy/cautery (total area <2 cm per week), refer for laser.
- *Exophytic cervical* – colposcopy and biopsy.
- *Oral* – refer to oral surgeon.
- No treatment is an option in any site, especially in vaginal and anal canal.

Pregnancy

- Podophyllin/otoxin, Imiquimod not approved for use.
- Warts often multiply in second and third trimester; treatment aims to reduce number of lesions present at delivery (risk of infant laryngeal papillomas +/− anogenital warts).

Cervical cytology

The NHS cervical screening programme recommends that no changes are required to screening intervals in women with anogenital warts.

Follow-up

- If new lesions evolving and original lesions have responded well, continue with current regime.
- Under 50% response/not tolerating treatment, consider change in regime.

Management

- Condom use may prevent transmission to uninfected partner.
- Be aware of psychological impact; refer for counselling if appropriate.
- Document cervical cytology; colposcopy if macroscopic cervical warts present.

Sexual partners

- Examine, screen and counsel.
- May be useful to contact trace in order to get sexual partners to attend for opportunistic screening.

Gonorrhoea (GC) (Females: uncomplicated)

Background

Gonorrhoea (GC) is the clinical disease resulting from infection with the Gram-negative diplococcus *Neisseria gonorrhoeae*. The primary sites of infection are the mucous membranes of the urethra, endocervix, rectum, pharynx and conjunctiva. Transmission is by direct inoculation of infected secretions from one mucous membrane to another.

Neisseria gonorrhoeae may co-exist with other genital mucosal pathogens, notably *Trichomonas vaginalis*, *Candida albicans* and *Chlamydia trachomatis*. If symptoms are present, they may be attributable to the co-infecting pathogen.

Incubation

The incubation period is 3–5 days.

Symptoms

- Frequently asymptomatic (up to 50%).
- Vaginal discharge.
- Lower abdominal pain.
- Pharyngeal usually asymptomatic (>90%).

Signs

- Occasional muco-purulent cervical discharge.
- Pelvic tenderness.
- Often normal appearance.

Diagnosis

- Microscopy of Gram stain to see Gram-negative intracellular diplococci from urethra, cervix +/− ano rectum.
- Culture from urethra, cervix +/− ano rectum +/− pharynx.
- Antigen detection tests are available (NAAT).
- If positive on antigen detection, culture to be performed to determine antimicrobial sensitivity.

Treatment

Antimicrobial therapy should take account of local patterns of antimicrobial sensitivity to *N gonorrhoeae*. The chosen regimen should eliminate infection in at least 95% of those presenting in the local community. Refer to the local department of sexual health and microbiology to determine first-line therapy in your locality.

Gonorrhoea

Drug	Formulation	Dosage	Frequency	Duration
Ampicillin/	Oral tablets	2 g/3 g	Stat	
Amoxicillin +		1 g		
Probenecid*				
Ciprofloxacin*	Oral tablets	500 mg	Stat	
Ceftriaxone (current	IM	250 mg	Stat	
drug of choice)				
Cefixime	Oral tablets	400 mg	Stat	
Spectinomycin	IM	2 g	Stat	

*Where regional prevalence of penicillin-resistant *N gonorrhoeae* is ≤5%.

Lactam allergy

Spectinomycin 2 g IM as a single dose or ciprofloxacin 500 mg orally as a single dose when the infection is known or anticipated to be quinolone sensitive.

Pregnancy

Pregnant women should not be treated with quinolone or tetracycline antimicrobials.

Epidemiological treatment of chlamydia

Ideally, all patients with gonorrhoea should be treated presumptively for chlamydia as co-existing infection can occur in up to 25% of patients. Combining effective antimicrobial therapy against *C trachomatis* with single-dose therapy for gonococcal infection is particularly appropriate when there is doubt that a patient will return for follow-up evaluation.

Follow-up

- TOC at minimum three days post-treatment if by culture, or two weeks post-treatment if by an NAAT.
- Check compliance, sexual abstinence and partner notification.
- Issue contact slip(s).

Sexual partners

- Females diagnosed with B1 and symptomatic should contact trace within preceding two weeks or last reported sexual partner.

- Asymptomatic or B1 at other sites, contact trace up to preceding three months.
- Examine for STIs.
- Offer epidemiological treatment.

Complications

- PID.
- Bartholin's abscess.
- Systemic infection.
- Reactive arthritis.

Gonorrhoea (GC) (Males: uncomplicated)

Incubation

The incubation period is 3–5 days.

Symptoms

- Urethral discharge (80%), dysuria (50%).
- Dysuria, rectal pain and discharge.
- Asymptomatic <10%.
- Pharyngeal usually asymptomatic (>90%).

Signs

- Urethral discharge.
- Meatitis, proctitis.
- Often normal appearance.

Diagnosis

- Microscopy of Gram stain to see Gram-negative intracellular diplococci from urethra +/– ano rectum.
- Culture from urethra +/– ano rectum +/– pharynx.
- Antigen detection tests are available (NAAT).
- If positive on antigen detection, culture to be performed to determine antimicrobial sensitivity).

Treatment

See Gonorrhoea (Females).

Epidemiological treatment of chlamydia

See Gonorrhoea (Females).

Follow-up

See Gonorrhoea (Females).

Sexual partners

- Males diagnosed with B1 and symptomatic should contact trace within proceeding two weeks or last reported sexual partner.
- Asymptomatic or B1 at other sites, contact trace up to preceding three months.
- Examine for STIs.
- Offer epidemiological treatment.

Complications

- Epididymitis.
- Balanitis.
- Reactive arthritis.

Hepatitis A (HAV)

Background

Hepatitis A (HAV) is caused by a picorna (RNA) virus. It is particularly common in areas of the world where sanitation is poor and mainly affects children. In the developed world it is less common; when it does occur it can be in any age group.

Transmission

- Faeco-oral (via food, water, close personal contact).
- Outbreaks have been reported in men who have sex with men, linked to oro-anal or digital-rectal contact, multiple sexual partners, anonymous partners, sex in public places and group sex.
- HIV-positive patients are not at increased risk but may be more infectious.
- In HIV-positive patients, hepatitis A viraemia may continue for over 90 days.
- Outbreaks have also been reported among intravenous drug users, in institutions for people with learning difficulties, and in contaminated batches of factor VIII.
- Patients are infectious for approximately two weeks before and one week after the jaundice by the non-parenteral routes, but virus can be found in the blood and stool until after the serum amino-transferase levels have peaked.

Incubation

The incubation period is 15–45 days. The infectious period is from two weeks before the onset of jaundice, and up to one week afterwards.

Symptoms

- Jaundice.
- Pale stools.
- Dark urine.
- Liver enlargement/tenderness.
- Dehydration.
- Asymptomatic in up to 50% of adults.

Vaccination: who to consider

- Homosexual/bisexual men.
- Haemophiliacs.
- Sexual/household contacts of HAV-positive individual.
- Those travelling to developing countries.
- Occupational exposure.
- IVDUs.
- Chronic hepatitis C sufferers.

Vaccination schedule	Protection	Follow-up
0, 6, 12 months	95% protection for at least 5 years	Revaccinate after 10 years
		Reduced response in immuno-compromised patients

- Combined hepatitis A and B vaccine can be given on the same schedule as hepatitis B vaccine. Early immunity to hepatitis B may be impaired.

Hepatitis B (HBV)

Background

Hepatitis B (HBV) is caused by a hepadna (DNA) virus. Hepatitis B is endemic worldwide, apart from isolated communities, with very high carriage rates (up to 20%) particularly in South and East Asia, but also in southern Europe, Central and South America, Africa and eastern Europe.

Transmission

- Sexual transmission occurs in unvaccinated or non-immune men who have sex with men and correlates with multiple partners, unprotected anal sex and oro-anal sex ('rimming').
- Transmission also occurs after heterosexual contact.
- Sex workers are also at higher risk.
- Parenteral (blood, blood products, drug users sharing needles and syringes, needle-stick, acupuncture).

- Vertical (infected mother to infant).
- Sporadic infection occurs in people without apparent risk factors, in institutions for learning difficulties and also in children in countries of high endemicity, but in these cases the means of transmission is poorly understood.

Incubation

The incubation period is 40–160 days. The infectious period is from two weeks before the onset of jaundice until the client becomes surface antigen negative.

Symptoms

Asymptomatic in 10–50% of adults.
    Possible symptoms are:

- Jaundice.
- Fatigue.
- Abdominal pain.

- Loss of appetite.
- Nausea, vomiting.
- Joint pain.

Diagnosis

Hepatitis B serology diagnosis table

Stage of infection	Surface antigen (HBsAG)	'e' antigen (HBeAG)	IgM anti-core body (HBc)	IgG anti-core antibody (HBc)	Hepatitis B virus DNA	Anti HBe	Anti HBs (HB surface)
Acute (early)	+	+	+	+	+	−	−
Acute (resolving)	+	−	+	+	−	+/−	−
Chronic (high activity)	+	+/−	−	+	+	+/−	−
Chronic (low infectivity)	+	−	−	+	−	+/−	−
Resolved (immune)	−	−	−	+	−	+/−	+/−
Successful vaccination	−	−	−	−	−	−	+

Vaccination: who to consider

- Homosexual/bisexual men.
- IVDUs.
- Sex workers of either sex.
- HIV-infected people.

- Survivors of sexual assault.
- Sexual assault victims.
- Sexual/household contacts of HBV-positive individual.
- People from/travelling to high prevalence areas (not western Europe, North America and Australasia).
- Needle-stick victims.
- Those with hepatitis C or other liver disease.
- Those with partners from high-risk groups.
- Occupational risk.

Markers	Significance
Anti HBc	Past exposure to hepatitis B (with neg HBsAG)
	Chronic hepatitis B (with pos HBsAG)
HBsAG	Acute or chronic hepatitis B carriage
Anti HBs	Immunity to hepatitis B
IgM anti HBc	Acute hepatitis B
	Chronic hepatitis B (low titre)
HBeAG	Acute or chronic hepatitis B
	Indicates continued infectious state
Anti HBe	Resolving acute hepatitis B
	Chronic hepatitis B (low risk)

Vaccination

Response to initial vaccine = blood titre level of 10 to >100 IU/l

- HIV-positive patients show reduced response rates to vaccination and become anti-HB surface negative more quickly.
- Test titre levels 4–12 weeks post last vaccination course.
- Give poor responders up to three repeat injections. Also consider PRE S vaccine.
- Evidence suggests that if vaccine courses are not completed by immuno-competent individuals, outstanding doses can be given four or more years later without need to restart three-dose course.
- One dose = 40% immunity; two doses = 90% immunity.
- It is probable that booster doses of vaccine are not required for at least 15 years in the immuno-competent who have responded to the initial vaccine (adults and children).
- HIV-positive and other immuno-compromised patients will need to be monitored and given booster doses if anti-HBs levels fall below 100 IU/l.

Vaccination schedule	Advantages	Disadvantages
0, 7, 21 days, 12 months (over 18-year-olds) 65.2% and 76% of vaccines having protective antibodies within one and five weeks respectively following third dose. One month after fourth dose 98.6% vaccines achieved protective antibody levels	• Rapid immunity • Short duration • High antibody titres at 12 and 13 months • Potential for better uptake	• Not tested in immuno-compromised • Little published data • Low titres in first year but evidence suggests protection adequate in immuno-competent
0, 1, 2, 12 months 15% and 89% of vaccines having protective antibodies one month after first dose and one month after third dose respectively. One month after the fourth dose 95.8% of vaccines achieved protective antibody levels	• Early immunity • High antibody titres at 12 and 13 months • Shorter time to early immunity than below	• Antibody levels lower than below in first year
0, 1, 6 months	• Higher antibody titres at 7 months • Long-established regimen	• Mostly researched in HIV • Poor 6/12-dose uptake

Discussion around accepted titre level that deems effective immunity should be had with your local virology department. It may vary according to locality and what evidence basis is being used as a definition.

Hepatitis C (HCV)

Background

Hepatitis C (HCV) is an RNA virus in the *Flaviviridae* family. Hepatitis C is endemic worldwide with high prevalence rates in South and East Asia and eastern Europe.

Transmission

- Parenteral spread accounts for the majority of cases through shared needles/syringes in intravenous drug users (IVDUs).
- Transfusion of blood or blood products (pre-1990s).
- Renal dialysis.
- Needle-stick injury or sharing a razor with an infected individual.
- Sexual transmission occurs at a low rate (approximately 0.2–2% per year of relationship, or 1–11% of partners in long-term relationships) but these rates increase if the index patient is also HIV infected.

There is an increased rate of carriage for:

- men who have sex with men attending GU clinics, but this is largely linked to HIV co-infection

- female sex workers
- former prisoners
- tattoo recipients and alcoholics
- IVDUs
- haemophiliacs*
- needle-stick injury
- sexual contacts
- individuals with hepatitis B or with liver disease
- vertical spread also occurs at a low rate (5% or less in most studies), but higher rates (up to 40%) are seen if the woman is both HIV and HCV.[3]

*Since 1990 all donated blood in the UK has been screened for HCV, and all blood products rendered incapable of transmitting infection.

Incubation

The incubation period is 4–20 weeks. Infectious period two weeks before onset of jaundice. Blood test can need a period of 3–9 months before detection.

Symptoms

Asymptomatic in >80% of adults.

Herpes simplex virus (HSV)

Background

- Herpes simplex virus type 1(HSV-1, the usual cause of oro-labial herpes) or herpes simplex virus type 2 (HSV-2).
- Following primary infection, the virus becomes latent in local sensory ganglia, periodically reactivating to cause symptomatic lesions or asymptomatic, but infectious, viral shedding. Infection may be primary or non-primary. Disease episodes may be initial or recurrent and symptomatic or asymptomatic.
- Prior infection with HSV-1 modifies the clinical manifestations of first infection by HSV-2.
- After childhood, symptomatic primary infection with HSV-1 is equally likely to be acquired in the genital area or oral areas.
- The majority of individuals found to have asymptomatic HSV-2 infections subsequently develop symptomatic lesions.

Primary/first episode HSV

Incubation period

The incubation period is 3–10 days, maybe longer.

Symptoms

- Painful ulcers.
- Blisters.
- Dysuria.
- Vaginal or urethral discharge.
- Often preceded by flu-like symptoms (more common in primary infections).
- Local irritation.
- May be asymptomatic and disease unrecognised.

Signs

- Blistering and ulceration of external genitalia +/− cervix and/or rectum.
- Lymphadenopathy.

Diagnosis

- Clinical.
- Viral culture swab.
- Serology test is available but is not type specific.
- NB: patient's immune response can take 8–12 weeks to develop.
- All patients with genital ulceration should have syphilis serology.

Treatment

Within five days of initial attack or new lesion, antiviral therapy does not alter the natural history of the disease; topical is less effective than oral.

No benefit from combined oral and topical. No evidence for courses longer than five days though treatment may be continued if new lesions are still appearing.

HSV

Drug	Formulation	Dosage	Frequency	Duration
Aciclovir	Cream	200 mg	5× day	5 days
Valaciclovir	Tablet	500 mg	2× day	5 days

See *BNF* for other recommendations if above not applicable.

Management

- Supportive – EMLA cream or lignocaine gel, petroleum jelly, salt-water baths, analgesia.
- Discussion – counselling should include: natural history, asymptomatic viral shedding (this is an important cause of transmission and is more common in HSV-2, in first year after infection and individual with frequent symptomatic recurrences), transmission risk (sexual and other means), and treatment options.

- Patients should abstain from sexual contact during lesion recurrences or prodromes.
- Teach recognition of recurrence.
- Efficacy of condoms not formally established.
- Failure to control everyday stressors does not affect recurrence.
- Hospitalisation may be indicated for urinary retention (suprapubic catheter), meningism, severe systemic symptoms or if intravenous therapy required.

Sexual partners

GU screen and counselling.

Recurrences

- Common, though lower with HSV-1; rates decline over time in most cases.
- Self-limiting and cause minor symptoms.

Complications

- Urinary retention.
- Sacral radiculopathy.
- Secondary bacterial infection.
- Aseptic meningitis.

Pregnancy

- Viral shedding incidence is high in pregnancy.
- First and second trimester acquisition – oral aciclovir in standard doses. (Not licensed for use in pregnancy but substantial clinical evidence supports its safety.)
- Aciclovir suppressive treatment from 34 weeks may reduce recurrence.
- Need for continuous aciclovir therapy and to consider Caesarean section (CS) in all women with primary episode developing within four weeks of delivery.
- Notify obstetric staff.

Refractory HSV lesions

These are lesions that do not respond to aciclovir treatment; consider whether the client is immuno-compromised.

Recurrent episode HSV

Symptoms

Less severe than initial presentation. Usually self-limiting.

Signs

See Primary HSV.

Diagnosis

See Primary HSV.

Treatment

- Depends on frequency, severity and relationship status.
- Patient-initiated treatment early in episode is most likely to be effective.
- Suppressive treatment more than six episodes/year – refer as appropriate.
- Should be discontinued after one year to assess recurrence frequency; assessment period should include two recurrences.
- Those with unacceptably high rates of recurrence may recommence suppressive treatment.

Follow-up

See Primary HSV.

Management

See Primary HSV.

Sexual partners

See Primary HSV.

Pregnancy

In recurrent HSV risk to foetus is small and is set against risk to mother of Caesarean section.

HIV/AIDS

Human immunodeficiency virus

Human immunodeficiency virus (HIV) attacks the body's immune system, making it hard to fight off infections. It targets specific white blood cells known as CD4 cells. The lower a person's CD4 count, the weaker their immune system will be.

Symptoms will vary enormously across individuals. Many will become infected and experience nothing. Weeks or months after exposure others will have a flu-like illness, develop a rash, have night sweats or more rarely have a life-threatening brain infection. All too often people coming for a test report vague symptoms similar to the above but eventually test negative. A blood test is therefore the only reliable means of detection.

Transmission

For someone to become infected, a sufficient amount of HIV must get into their blood. Body fluids which contain enough HIV to infect someone are blood, semen, vaginal fluids (including menstrual blood) and breast milk.

The main ways in the UK of passing HIV on to another person are as follows.

- Sex without a condom – HIV can pass from one person to another through unprotected anal or vaginal sex. A small risk exists with oral sex.
- Injecting drug use – HIV can be passed on by using needles or syringes and other injecting equipment that someone with HIV has already used.
- Mother to baby – a pregnant woman may pass the virus to her baby before or during birth, or HIV can be passed on during breastfeeding.
- Organ transplant, blood transfusion or blood products – since 1985, all blood and tissue donations and blood products in the UK have been screened for HIV.

There is no cure or vaccine for HIV. Some powerful anti-HIV drugs are available. Taking these in various combinations can slow down the damage HIV does to the immune system.

Acquired immune deficiency syndrome (AIDS)

An HIV-damaged immune system leaves a person open to other illnesses, e.g. tuberculosis, pneumonia and cancers. Once diagnosed with such an illness the person is often said to have AIDS. It is a term falling out of use. Instead it is increasingly called 'late stage' or 'advanced HIV infection'.

The process of HIV testing

The following guidance is taken from procedures in our service. In developing these procedures we have closely referred to the Department of Health (DoH) guidelines for pretest discussion on HIV testing[4] and the BASHH draft guidance on HIV testing 2004.[5]

HIV testing is becoming a normalised and standard test – the aim being to destigmatise and demystify the test and the infection.

The discussion about HIV and HIV testing should now be part of mainstream clinical care. Specialist counsellors may be required if the circumstances of the individual attending for HIV testing are complex and time consuming and further discussion is required.

It must be noted that the principles of this section are transferable when dealing with other STIs.

General importance of the HIV test

The early detection of HIV infection by antibody testing may:

- allow the individual to obtain immediate optimum medical and supportive healthcare

- allow the individual to receive counselling and advice and take action to prevent transmission
- allow women who may have been infected to seek advice and make decisions about conception, the management of pregnancy and breastfeeding
- allow the individual to protect their sexual partners from the risk of infection
- allow the collection of information on the spread of the epidemic which assists prevention and service planning
- allow partner notification.

The HIV discussion

There are five main components of pre-test discussion:

1 ensuring the individual understands the nature of HIV infection; provision of information about HIV transmission and risk reduction
2 a discussion of risk activities the individual may have been involved in with respect to HIV infection, including the date of the last risk activity and the perception of the need for a test
3 discussion of the benefits and difficulties to the individual, his or her family and associates of having a test and knowing the result whether positive or negative
4 giving details of the test and how the result will be provided
5 obtaining an informed decision about whether or not to proceed with the test.

Indications for testing

- Unprotected sexual practice.
- History of drug use and especially injecting exposure.
- History of exposure to blood/blood production transfusion, particularly prior to screening of donations and heat treatment of factor VIII.
- Occupational risk.
- Overseas travel with exposure to high-risk activity.

If the individual is diagnosed as HIV-positive the health professional should:

- address the patient's immediate reactions
- refer for specialist management, including treatment where appropriate
- give details of support services
- offer follow-up appointments and ongoing support, which may include addressing issues concerned with legal matters and support for carers and partners.

Treatment

Treatment for HIV is a highly specialised area that is rapidly changing. Referral to a specialist centre would always be the route for an individual testing positive.

Lymphogranuloma venereum (LGV)

Background

Lymphogranuloma venereum (LGV) is a systemic disease caused by one of three invasive serovars L1, L2, or L3 of *Chlamydia trachomatis*, but other strains may occasionally be involved.

Clinical features

The clinical course of LGV is classically divided into three stages:

- primary lesions
- secondary lesions
- genito-ano-rectal syndrome.

Long-term complications

- The destruction of lymph nodes may result in lymphoedema of genitals (elephantiasis).
- An association with rectal cancer has been reported; certainly the two conditions can be confused and a differential diagnosis may be necessary.

The recent outbreak of LGV is among gay men who present with proctitis. So far most men are HIV-positive. All cases to date have been with serotype L2.

Symptoms

Presentation is usually with one of two syndromes:

- *Ano-rectal syndrome.* In the recent outbreak proctitis is the most usual presentation. Symptoms include anal discharge, pain and tenesmus. All gay men with rectal symptoms should be offered rectal chlamydia testing. There may also be fever, diarrhoea, and abdominal pain and abscess formation.
- *Inguinal syndrome.* Painful inguinal adenopathy – bubo genital or anal ulcers (usually small and transient, can be large and painful in HIV co-infected patients). Systemic symptoms (fever, malaise, etc.) often present.

See www.bashh.org or www.hpa.org.uk for further guidance on the treatment and management of the infection.

Molluscum

Background

Molluscum contagiosum is caused by a pox virus. The virus is probably passed on by direct skin-to-skin contact, and may affect any part of the body. Sexual contact may lead to the appearance of lesions in the genital area. There is anecdotal evidence associating facial lesions with HIV-related immunodeficiency.

Incubation

The incubation period is three to 12 weeks.

Symptoms

- Pearly, papular, smooth or umbilicated lesions.
- In immunocompetent individuals, their size does not usually exceed 5 mm, and if untreated they usually regress spontaneously after several months.

Diagnosis

Based on characteristic appearance.

Treatment

Molluscum

Cryotherapy
Podophyllotoxin cream 0.5%
Imiquimod cream 5%

- Aim of treatment is tissue destruction.
- Cryotherapy – repeat applications may be necessary.
- Expression of the pearly core, either manually or using forceps.
- Piercing with an orange stick (with/without the application of phenol or iodine).
- Curettage or diathermy under local anaesthetic.
- Podophyllotoxin cream 0.5% can be self-applied.
- Imiquimod cream 5% can be self-applied (unlicensed use in the UK).

Pregnancy and breastfeeding

- Cryotherapy and other, purely mechanical methods of destruction are safe.
- Podophyllotoxin should not be used.

Follow-up

No specific follow-up is indicated.

Management

Offer full GU screen.

Sexual partners

- No specific need for contact tracing.
- Examine for STIs.

Non-gonococcal urethritis/non-specific urethritis

Background

Urethritis, or inflammation of the urethra, is a multifactoral condition which is primarily sexually acquired. It is characterised by discharge and/or dysuria but may be asymptomatic. *Chlamydia trachomatis* is the commonest cause of non-gonococcal urethritis (NGU), accounting for 30–50% of cases. *Ureaplasma urealyticum* (ureaplasmas) and *Mycoplasma genitalium* probably cause urethritis and account for 10% and 20% of cases respectively. *Trichomonas vaginalis* has been reported in 1–17% of cases of NGU. It is likely that the relative importance of *T vaginalis* as a cause of NGU depends on the prevalence of the infection within the community. *N meningitidis*, herpes simplex virus, candida, bacterial urinary tract infection, urethral stricture and foreign bodies probably account for only a small proportion of cases (<10%). There is also a possible association with bacterial vaginosis. Between 20% and 30% of men with NGU have no organism detected. Asymptomatic urethritis, without an observable discharge, may have a different aetiology from symptomatic urethritis, with *C trachomatis* being detected less frequently.

It is assumed that the aetiological agent of sexually acquired male NGU could potentially cause genital tract inflammation in women, in particular pelvic inflammatory disease (PID). This is unquestionably the case with chlamydial and gonococcal infection but remains to be substantiated for other causes. However, as the aetiology of PID is unknown in 40–60% of cases, this assumption remains a possibility.

Incubation

The incubation period is 14–21 days (often a few months into a new relationship).

Symptoms

- Asymptomatic.
- Urethral discharge.
- Dysuria.
- Penile irritation.

Signs

- Often normal appearance.
- Urethral inflammation and discharge (this may only be present on urethral massage).

Diagnosis

- Gram stain ≤5 polymorphs/high power field from urethral smear
  and/or
- Gram stain from a first-pass urine (FPU) specimen ≥10 polymorphs/high power field from threads. Urine to have been held for more than four hours.

Symptomatic clients, in whom no urethritis is detected, should be asked to return the following day having held their urine for at least four to six hours.

Treat empirically if observable mucopurulent or purulent discharge/at high risk of infection/unlikely to return.

Treatment

NGU

Drug	Formulation	Dosage	Frequency	Duration
Doxycycline	Oral tablet	100 mg	bd	7 days
Azithromycin	Oral tablet	1 g	Stat	

Follow-up

- At seven days, check compliance, sexual abstinence and partner notification.
- A repeat urethral smear and FPU is *only* indicated in clients who remain symptomatic or have a urethral discharge on examination.
- If urethritis ≥5 polymorphs at follow-up, consider re-prescribing first-line treatment plus metronidazole 400 mg oral bd for five days.
- If symptoms/signs persist despite above, refer as appropriate.

Management

- Advise no sex or unprotected sex until follow-up appointment.
- Issue contact slip(s).
- Offer full GU screen.

Asymptomatic men

Issue contact slips to client to give to sexual partner(s) in last six months, or last other sexual partner, whichever is the longer time period.

Symptomatic men

Issue contact slip(s) to sexual partners over last four weeks or for the duration of symptoms.

Sexual partners

- Examine for STIs.
- Offer epidemiological treatment.

Complications

- Conjunctivitis.
- Epididimo-orchitis.
- Sexually acquired reactive arthritis (SARA).

Treatment

Refer as appropriate.

Pelvic inflammatory disease (PID)

Background

Pelvic inflammatory disease (PID) is usually the result of infection ascending from the endocervix causing endometritis, salpingitis, parametritis, oophoritis, tubo-ovarian abcess and/or pelvic peritonitis. *Neisseria gonorrhoeae* and *Chlamydia trachomatis* have been identified as causative agents, while *Gardnerella vaginalis*, anaerobes and other organisms commonly found in the vagina may also be implicated. *Mycoplasma genitalium* has also been associated with upper genital tract infection in women.

PID may be symptomatic or asymptomatic. Even when present, clinical symptoms and signs lack sensitivity and specificity.

Symptoms

(Suggestive of PID)

- Lower abdominal pain.
- Dyspareunia.
- Abnormal bleeding.
- Abnormal vaginal/cervical discharge.

Signs

- Lower abdominal tenderness.
- Adnexal tenderness on bimanual vaginal examination.
- Cervical excitation.
- Fever (>38°C).

Diagnosis

- Clinical diagnosis 65–90% compared to laparoscopy diagnosis.
- High index of suspicion in women with lower genital tract infection.

- Elevated ESR (erythrocyte sedimentation rate) or C reactive protein.
- The absence of documented infection in the genital tract does not exclude PID.
- Screen for chlamydia and gonorrhoea.

Differential diagnosis

- Ectopic pregnancy, acute appendicitis, endometriosis, complications of ovarian cyst, functional pain.
- Assess severity of disease clinically, i.e. mild, moderate and severe.

Treatment

Broad-spectrum antibiotic therapy is required to cover *N gonorrhoeae*, *C trachomatis* and a variety of aerobic and anaerobic bacteria commonly isolated from the upper genital tract in women with PID.

PID

Drug	Formulation	Dosage	Frequency	Duration
Ceftriaxone	IM	250 mg	Stat	
Ciprofloxacin	Oral tablets	500 mg	Stat	
Doxycycline	Oral tablets	100 mg	bd	14 days
Metronidazole	Oral tablets	400 mg	bd	10 days
Pregnancy risk:				
Amoxicillin	Oral tablets	3 g	Stat	
Erythromycin	Oral tablets	500 mg	bd	14 days
Metronidazole	Oral tablets	400 mg	bd	10 days

Follow-up

- Review in 72 hours to monitor clinical response.
- If clinical improvement review again at two weeks.
- Further review at four weeks recommended, reviewing clinical response, compliance and contact tracing.
- Refer to health adviser at diagnosis/follow-up as appropriate.

Management

- Pregnancy test.
- IUD *in situ* – consider removal in clinically severe PID.
- Mild disease – treat. Moderate disease – treat and refer. Severe or diagnosis in doubt – refer urgently.

Sexual partners

- Examine for STIs especially chlamydia and gonorrhoea.
- Offer epidemiological treatment for chlamydia and gonorrhoea.

- No unprotected sex until therapy completed and partner(s) tested/treated.
- Issue contact slips to client to give to relevant sexual partner(s) within six months of onset of symptoms or last other sexual partner (whichever is the longer time period).

Complications

- Fitz-Hugh syndrome (right upper quadrant pain in association with perihepatitis) in 10–20% women with PID.
- Women with HIV may have more severe symptoms.

Pubic lice or crabs (*Pediculosis pubis*)

Background

The crab louse *Pthirus pubis* is transmitted by close body contact. The incubation period is usually between five days and several weeks, although occasional individuals appear to have more prolonged, asymptomatic infestation.

Incubation

The incubation period is 5 to 28 days.

Symptoms

- Itching of pubic/perianal area.
- Can be asymptomatic.
- May involve other sites (e.g. axillae, eyelashes and eyebrows).
- Blue macules (maculae caeruleae), may be visible at feeding sites.

Signs

Pubic lice ('crabs') and 'nits'.

Diagnosis

- Identification of 'crabs' and 'nits'/eggs (magnifying glass can be used).
- Examination under light microscope can confirm the exact morphology if necessary.

Treatment

Pthirus pubis infection

Malathion 0.5% cream
Permethrin 1% cream rinse

- Head lice may develop resistance to pediculicides.
- Lotions are likely to be more effective than shampoos, and should be applied to all body hair including the beard and moustache if necessary.
- Shaving of pubic hair unnecessary.

Infested eyelashes

- Permethrin 1% lotion, with eyelashes closed.
- Application of Vaseline/removal by forceps.

Follow-up

- At one week to re-examine for the absence of lice.
- Eggs may be found some time after successful treatment.
- Second application after 3–7 days may be advisable. Consider alternative treatment from above list.

Sexual partners

- Avoid close bodily contact.
- Treat sexual contacts over the previous three months. Give contact slip(s).
- Examine for STIs.
- Give epidemiological treatment.

Pregnancy/breastfeeding

Permethrin or malathion 0.5% (aqueous cream) is the agent of choice in pregnancy, due to poor absorption and rapid metabolism by the body after topical application. Aqueous preparations are preferable to alcohol preparations.

Scabies (*Sarcoptes scabiei*)

Background

The infestation is caused by the mite *Sarcoptes scabiei*. Any part of the body may be affected, and transmission is by skin-to-skin contact.

Incubation

The incubation period is four to six weeks.

Symptoms

- Itchy rash (especially at night), sparing head and neck sites.
- Hypersensitivity reaction to mite excrement as they burrow under the skin to lay their eggs.

Signs

- Burrows/papules – can affect genital area.
- Silvery lines classically between fingers, wrists and elbows.
- HIV – crusted lesions which teem with mites (Norwegian scabies).

Diagnosis

Clinical appearance is usually typical; scraping from burrows examined under the light microscope.

Treatment

Scabies

Permethrin 5% cream
Malathion 0.5% aqueous lotion

Follow-up

Re-treat only if new burrows seen.

Management

- Wash linen/clothes >50°C if possible. Mites separated from the human host die after 72 hours.
- Avoid body contact until treated and followed up.

Sexual partners

- Consider institutional/household contacts.
- Treat sexual contacts over the previous two months. Give contact slip(s).
- Examine for STIs.
- Give epidemiological treatment.

Pregnancy/breastfeeding

Permethrin or malathion 0.5% (aqueous cream) is the agent of choice in pregnancy, due to poor absorption and rapid metabolism by the body after topical application. Aqueous preparations are preferable to alcohol preparations.

Syphilis – early (primary, secondary, early latent)

Background

Syphilis is classified as acquired or congenital. Acquired syphilis is divided into:

- early (primary, secondary and early latent <2 years of infection)
- late (late latent >2 years, tertiary including gummatous, cardiovascular and neurological involvement).

Congenital syphilis is divided into:

- early (first two years)
- late (including stigmata of congenital syphilis).

Primary syphilis

- Characteristed by an ulcer (the chancre) and regional lymphadenopathy. The chancre is classically in the anogenital region, single, painless and indurated with a clean base discharging clear serum.
- Chancres may be atypical: multiple, painful, purulent and destructive, may cause the syphilitic balanitis of Follman, and may be extragenital.
- There may also be a mixed aetiology. Any anogenital ulcer should be considered to be syphilitic or herpetic unless proven otherwise. Herpetic ulcers may be atypical.
- Chancroid, lymphogranuloma venereum and donovanosis should be considered if the ulcer is acquired in the tropics.

Secondary syphilis

- Characterised by multisystem involvement within the first two years of infection: generalised polymorphic rash often affecting the palms and soles, condylomata lata, mucocutaneous lesions, generalised lymphadenopathy; less commonly, patchy alopecia, meningitis, cranial nerve palsies, hepatitis, splenomegaly and glomerulonephritis.
- The rash is classically non-itchy but may be itchy, particularly in dark-skinned patients.

Early latent syphilis

- Characterised by positive serological tests for syphilis with no clinical evidence of treponemal infection within the first two years of infection.

HIV and syphilis

- Newly diagnosed syphilis patients should have an HIV test done; early syphilis may increase risk of HIV acquisition. HIV transmission risk may be increased in those with positive syphilis diagnosis.
- HIV concomitant infection may affect the natural history of syphilis and cause unusual manifestations or reactivation of previously treated disease.
- Treatment is with higher doses of penicillin for longer duration.

In the UK an EIA test is generally performed to determine if a patient has an immunological response to having come into contact with the treponeme responsible for syphilis infection. If the EIA is positive then the following tests are performed to further confirm initial reaction and/or clarify stage of infection. Further guidance on syphilis diagnosis can be sought from the Health Protection Agency at: www.hpa.org.uk/cdph/issues/CDPHvol3/No3/guidelines.pdf.

Syphilis serology interpretation table

	VDRL (RPR)	TPHA	FTA
Very early syphilis	−	−	−
Primary syphilis	+/− or +	−	+
Secondary syphilis	High titre +	+	+
Latent or yaws	Low titre +/−	+	+
Treated syphilis	− or weak +	+	+
Biological false positive	+	−	−

Please refer to national guidance at www.bashh.org/guidelines.asp or the *BNF* for guidance on current recommended drug therapy, or refer to your local department of GU medicine.

Trichomonas vaginalis (TV)

Background

Trichomonas vaginalis (TV) is a flagellated protozoan. In women the organism is found in the vagina, urethra and paraurethral glands. While the urinary tract is the sole site of infection in less than 5% of cases, urethral infection is present in 90% of episodes. In men infection is usually of the urethra, although trichomonas has been isolated from the subpreputial sac and lesions of the penis.

In adults transmission is almost exclusively sexually transmitted. Due to site specificity, infection can only follow intravaginal or intraurethral inoculation of the organism.

Symptoms

Females

- Offensive vaginal discharge.
- Vulval itching.
- Dysuria.
- 10–50% asymptomatic.
- Occasional lower abdominal pain.

Males

- 15–50% asymptomatic.
- Urethral discharge.

- Dysuria, frequency.
- Rarely prostatitis.

Signs

Females

- Up to 70% vaginal discharge (frothy yellow discharge in 10–30% of women).
- Vulvitis/vaginitis.
- 2% strawberry cervix to naked eye.
- 5–15% no abnormalities found.

Males

- 50–60% men urethral discharge.
- No signs.
- Rarely balanoposthitis.

Diagnosis

Females

- Observe on wet smear, specimen taken from posterior fornix (diagnose 40–80% cases).
- Culture media (diagnose up to 95%).

NB: Trichomonads can be diagnosed on cytology (60–80%), but 30% are false positives. To be confirmed by observation of vaginal discharge + culture.

Males

- Observation by wet mount of specimen (up to 30% cases).
- Urethral culture or culture first-void urine (60–80% cases).
- Detection significantly increased if both done together.

Treatment

TV

Drug	Formulation	Dosage	Frequency	Duration
Metronidazole	Oral tablets	2 g 400–500 mg	Stat bd	5–7 days

Follow-up

Test of cure to be undertaken if symptomatic post-treatment or if symptoms recur.

Management

- GU screen.
- No sexual intercourse until TOC.
- Issue contact slips.

Sexual partners

- Routine screening and epidemiological treatment of sexual partners.
- Male contact of TV found to have NGU – treat first for TV, then repeat urethral smear at follow-up before additionally treating for NGU.

Pregnancy and breastfeeding

- Associated with preterm delivery/low birth weight.
- Treat with oral metronidazole as indicated.

NB:
- Stat doses of metronidazole contraindicated in pregnancy.
- Symptoms in early pregnancy – clotrimazole pessary 100 mg od seven days or Aci-Jel can be used.

Recurrences/relapses

Refer as appropriate.

Complications

May enhance HIV transmission.

References

1 Department of Health (2000) *A Pilot Study of Opportunistic Screening for Genital Chlamydia Trachomatis Infection in England (1999–2000). Summary report.* DoH, London.
2 British Association of Sexual Health and HIV Clinical Effectiveness Group (2002) *National Guidelines on the Management of NGU.* www.bashh.org/guidelines/2002/ngu_090IC.pdf
3 National Institute for Clinical Excellence (2004) www.nice.org.uk/download.aspx?o=ta075publicinfo
4 Department of Health (1996) *Guidelines: pretest discussion for HIV.* www.dh.gov.uk/assetRoot/04/12/54/85/04125485.pdf
5 British Association of Sexual Health and HIV Clinical Effectiveness Group (2004) *Draft Guidance on HIV Testing.* www.bashh.org/guidelines/ceguidelines.htm

Chapter 13

Contact tracing

Contact tracing, or partner notification, has been defined as:

> The process of contacting the sexual partners of an individual with a sexually transmitted infection including HIV, and advising them that they have been exposed to infection. By this means, people who are at high risk of STI/HIV, many of whom are unaware that they have been exposed, are contacted and encouraged to attend for counselling, testing and other prevention and treatment services.[1]

Contact tracing or partner notification?

At the end of the 1980s the public healthcare establishment responded to political pressure by dropping the out-of-favour term 'contact tracing' and replacing it with 'partner notification'. It was felt that this took the emphasis away from the investigative nature of the practice and implied a more personal approach. There remained, however, a view that the one-dimensional activity of 'notifying' individuals of a potential exposure to infection undersold what is actually a far more complex activity.

The health adviser

This process has been traditionally carried out by health advisers in mainstream genito-urinary (GU) settings. With the growing availability of sexual health services in non-GU settings this genre of health professional is not always available. The process of partner notification is not therefore exclusive and should not be seen as such by anyone who will undertake the task. A definition of the process is below but, simplified, it is ensuring that the client whom you see understands that the infection they may have can ultimately contribute to many cycles of repeated infection in others, and that by notifying sexual contacts, these repeated cycles can potentially be halted.

Contact slips

These are issued by all GU services to patients wishing to notify their own contacts. The health professional may offer a contact slip, explaining how and why these are used:

- to give the contact sufficient information to book an appointment and find the service

- to enable the contact to be managed appropriately
- to inform the issuing clinic of the contact's attendance.

Content

- Clinic name, address, telephone number, opening times and location.
- Index patient number, diagnosis or diagnostic code and date of diagnosis.
- Contact details following presentation, including number, diagnosis, date of diagnosis and the name of the clinic.

There are differing opinions on whether or not the Kc60 code should be used, or whether the name of the diagnosed infection should be used in order to aid the demystification of the process. It will be down to local agreement and research to determine which method you will use. The overall aim is that, as practitioners, we effectively participate in the breaking of the chain of infection.

List of contact traceable infections

- Chancroid.
- Chlamydia.
- Genital warts.
- Gonorrhoea.
- Hepatitis A, B, C.
- HIV.
- NSU/NGU.
- Pubic lice.
- Scabies.
- Syphilis.
- Trichomoniasis.

Molluscum and genital herpes are not necessarily contact traced; in the case of herpes, psychological support may be required.

Reference

1 Crown F, French R and Johnson AM (1996) The role and effectiveness of partner notification in STD control: a review. *Genitourinary Medicine.* **72**: 247–52.

This section has closely referred to Chapter 1 in: Faldon C (2004) *The Manual for Sexual Health Advisers.* Society of Sexual Health Advisers, Amicus Health Sector, London. It can be accessed online at www.ssha.info/public/manual/index.asp

Chapter 14

Sexual assault

Sexual assault could easily be disclosed within a consultation, especially when asking about sexual coercion. When asking exploratory questions pertaining to abuse, coercion, grooming or assault, it is important to know exactly what you would do with that information.

If setting up services in a community setting and not a mainstream sexual health setting, there are restrictions as to what service you are able to provide. This is compounded by the fact that community-based services are likely to be sessional and, if catering for young people, the sessions are likely to occur primarily in the late afternoon or evening. This leaves the service in a somewhat isolated position with regards to accessing outside support services or agencies.

As a service, we have accommodated this scenario through the following provision: we have a counsellor and health adviser as part of our team, as well as a doctor who comes from a sexual assault background and have assigned a nurse to lead in that area for the service.

We have also ascertained what support services are in place that we can utilise effectively, the main ones being the Haven clinics or sexual assault referral centres (SARCs) around England who specialise in sexual assault and forensics.

A SARC is a one-stop location where victims of sexual assault can receive medical care and counselling while at the same time having the opportunity to assist the police investigation into alleged offences, and includes the facilities for a high standard of forensic examination.

Direct information about the SARCs can be gained from the following websites:

- www.thehavens.org.uk
- www.homeoffice.gov.uk.

Having such organisations in England has meant that the pressure to provide immediate clinical examination, testing and care to someone who discloses sexual assault can now be deferred to a specialist team, leaving community services able to focus on what other needs we can provide for as safely and effectively as the service allows. This could include areas such as:

- prophylactic antibiotic therapy
- two-week or more post-assault sexual health screening
- emergency contraception
- hepatitis/HIV screening and discussion
- counselling.

These are some of the things that need to be thought about when providing an integrated service. Examples of the sexual assault flowchart and telephone questionnaire used in our clinic are included as samples of practice in a community setting. Within a mainstream GU setting, processes, standards and pathways should be set locally or within a network.

Considerations within your service

Incubation period of common STIs

Sexually transmitted infection (STI)	Incubation period (days)
Neisseria gonorrhoeae	2–7
Herpes simplex virus	2–12
Trichomonas vaginalis	4–20
Chlamydia trachomatis	7–14
Treponema pallidum	14–84
Human immunodeficiency virus (HIV)	30–90
Human papilloma virus	30–140
Hepatitis B virus	45–180

Forensic evidence

Various types of forensic evidence may be available:

- semen
- seminal fluid
- saliva
- fibres
- blood
- hairs
- condom lubricant.

Immediate medical, psychological and social needs

- Emergency contraception.
- Prophylaxis against STIs (including hepatitis B and HIV).
- First aid for minor injuries.
- Investigation and treatment of more serious injuries.
- The support of a friend or family member.
- Replacement clothing (if still wearing the clothes worn at the time of the assault, as these will need to be retained).
- Safe accommodation.[1]

Lastly, you will need to consider guidelines specific to dealing with young people, especially those under 18 years, under 16 years and under 13 years old.

Recommended time to testing[2]

Tests	Presentation	Two weeks post-assault	One month post-presentation	Three months post-assault	Six months post-assault
Chlamydia	Recommended	If prophylaxis not given at first screen			
Gonorrhoea	Recommended	If prophylaxis not given at first screen			
Trichomonas or bacterial vaginosis	Recommended	If prophylaxis not given at first screen			
Syphilis	Recommended		If history or circumstance indicates	Recommended	
Serum save	Recommended				
HIV/hepatitis B abs	If history or circumstance indicates			Recommended	If history or circumstance indicates
Hepatitis C antibody	If history or circumstance indicates			If history or circumstance indicates	If history or circumstance indicates
Treatments: Postcoital contraception	If history or circumstance indicates				
Antibiotic prophylaxis	If history or circumstance indicates				
Hepatitis B vaccine	Recommended		Recommended	Recommended	
Counsellor review	Recommended	Recommended	If history or circumstance indicates	If history or circumstance indicates	If history or circumstance indicates

Guidance around provision of services for young people can be gained from the following places:

- Department of Health[3] (*see also* Chapter 8)
- www.bashh.org/guidelines/2002/adolescent_final_0903.pdf – also gives guidance on child drug treatment options for STIs and testing and clinical examination
- www.brook.org.uk
- www.homeoffice.gov.uk
- your local child protection team.

References

1 Rogers DJ (2002) Assisting and advising complainants of sexual assault in the family planning setting. *Journal of Family Planning and Reproductive Health Care.* **28**(3): 127–31.
2 BASHH (2001) *National Guidelines on the Management of Adult Victims of Sexual Assault.* Clinical Effectiveness Group. www.bashh.org/guidelines/2002/sexassault_0601.pdf
3 Department of Health (2004) *Best Practice Guidance for Doctors and Other Health Professionals on the Provision of Advice and Treatment to Young People Under 16 on Contraception, Sexual Health and Reproductive Health.* Department of Health, London.

Chapter 15

Formulary

This section closely refers to the Electronic Medicines Compendium (www. medicines.org.uk) and the British National Formulary 2005 (www.bnf.org/bnf/).

Prescribing today

This book is intended to be a desktop reference for any health professional working in the field of sexual and reproductive health; however, it was developed as a result of recent developments in prescribing for non-medical health professionals, who, as a result, can take on the holistic care of a client. This section will describe the recent legislation that has enabled health professionals other than doctors to supply drugs to clients through patient group directions, and prescribe through clinical management plans or as independent prescribers from specific formularies. It will also explain the differences between these methods of supplying or prescribing drugs.

Legislation

A number of pieces of legislation have been enacted in the last 35 years which work together to set a legislative framework for prescribing. The Medicines Act 1968 in UK legislation is the legal instrument that regulates the prescribing, supply and administration of medicines.[1] The legal framework for the supply of medicines to the general public is set out in the Act and in secondary legislation made under the Act, i.e. the Prescription Only Medicines Order 1997 and the Medicines (Pharmacy and General Sales – Exemption) Order 1980.[2,3] The Prescription Only Medicines Amendment Order Statutory Instrument 2003 no. 696 was the secondary legislation that brought forward supplementary prescribing.[4]

The Misuse of Drugs Act 1971 further controls the sale, supply and possession of substances that are liable to abuse.[5]

The Medicines Act and the Misuse of Drugs Act are part of the criminal law; breaches of these Acts render the person in breach liable to criminal prosecution. Both the police and the Pharmaceutical Society have the powers of prosecution under the Medicines Act.

The licensing of human medicines is handled by the Medicines and Healthcare products Regulatory Agency (MHRA) (previously the Medicines Control Agency). The Medicines Act set up a statutory advisory body called the Medicines Commission which in turn advises on the setting up of specialist advisory committees. The Committee on Safety of Medicines is one of these.

NHS regulations impose restrictions on the use of some medicines by professionals who are employed by or contract their services to the NHS. Breach of NHS regulations can affect an individual's employment status within the service.

The Medicinal Products Prescription by Nurses Act 1992[6] amended the Medicines Act 1968 and the NHS Act 1977[7] to allow nurses to prescribe. The Health and Social Care Act 2001 is the legal instrument that allows pharmacists and other healthcare professionals to prescribe.[8]

Legislation summary

Medicines Act 1968	Regulates the prescribing, supply and administration of medicines
NHS Act 1977	Contained guidance on prescribing in the NHS
Misuse of Drugs Act 1971	Controls the sale, supply and possession of substances that are liable to abuse
Medicines Order 1980 Prescription Only Medicines Order 1997	Secondary legislation to the Medicines Act
Medicinal Products Prescription by Nurses Act 1992	Amended Medicines Act and NHS Act to allow nurses to prescribe
Health and Social Care Act 2001	Legal instrument that allows pharmacists and other healthcare professionals to prescribe
Prescription Only Medicines Amendment Order 2003	Secondary legislation that brought forward supplementary prescribing

Independent nurse prescribing

District nurse and health visitor prescribers may currently prescribe medicines listed in the Nurse Practitioners' Formulary at the back of the British National Formulary (BNF).

In 2002, using the powers in the Medicinal Products Prescription by Nurses Act 1992, another subcategory of nurse was added to the list of practitioners who are allowed to prescribe. This group of nurses has been described as 'extended formulary or independent nurse prescribers'. Independent nurse prescribers can assess patients and prescribe medicines without reference to a doctor or a dentist, but the list of medicines they can prescribe is limited and can only be for medical conditions listed in the formulary.

The list of medicines that extended nurse prescribers can prescribe is published by the MHRA and can be found in current editions of the BNF.

The right to prescribe will be defined within a practitioner's job description, not by qualification alone.

Supplementary prescribing

Supplementary prescribing is a voluntary prescribing partnership between an independent prescriber and a supplementary prescriber to implement an agreed patient-specific clinical management plan (CMP) with the patient's agreement.

The criteria that are currently set in regulations for lawful supplementary prescribing are as follows.

- The independent prescriber must be a doctor or dentist.
- The supplementary prescriber must be a registered nurse, midwife or pharmacist (other healthcare professionals will be added in due course) who has attended and passed a validated prescribing course.
- The patient must agree to have their care transferred to another healthcare professional.
- There must be a written clinical management plan relating to a named patient and to that patient's specific conditions. Agreement to the plan must be recorded by both the independent and supplementary prescriber before supplementary prescribing begins.

Supplementary prescribers can prescribe for any condition, and prescribe any medicine that is not limited by previous NHS regulations. They can prescribe any Prescription-Only Medicine (POM), Pharmacy (P) or General Sales List (GSL) medicines provided they are within the CMP.

At present supplementary prescribers are not allowed to prescribe controlled drugs nor medicines that do not have a product licence and are not part of a clinical trial.

Patient group directions

A patient group direction (PGD) is a written direction, which must be signed by a doctor and a pharmacist, allowing supply and/or administration of a POM by authorised health professionals to patients without the need for a prescription. PGDs are documents that make it legal for medicines to be given to groups of patients without individual prescriptions having to be written for each patient.

Supply of medicines under a PGD is not a form of prescribing and there is no specific training that health professionals must undertake before they are able to work to a PGD.

The idea of PGDs came out of consideration by the Crown Review of Prescribing of what were known as 'group protocols', which were used mainly in hospitals to permit supply of medication to patients without the need for a specific prescription in every instance.[9] The Crown Review considered that these were unlawful and suggested an alternative method: patient group directions. Changes have been made to the Medicines Act 1968 to allow PGDs.

PGDs allow defined groups of healthcare professionals to supply medicines to treat specific medical conditions. Originally they were only for use within the NHS; however, in 2003 regulations were amended to permit the sale, supply or administration of medicines under PGDs in other specific non-NHS healthcare establishments.[10]

The field of nurse prescribing is constantly changing but as it stands presents a confusing picture both to those within healthcare and more so to patients and their families. For example, off-licence prescription of a medication would not be permissible through the ENPF (Extended Nurse Prescribers' Formulary) yet could be incorporated into a PGD.[11] Also the range of drugs available and the conditions outlined as treatable on the ENPF allow greater independence of practice in one area of nursing compared to another; for example, contraceptive nurse specialists can prescribe for all contraceptive methods and are only restricted in the newest of pills, whereas sexual health nurse specialists can prescribe for a restricted range of conditions and only with certain drugs – often these drugs are not first line or do not correspond with local resistance patterns and therefore are of little use.

General consensus among the nursing profession is that the BNF should be open to all trained nurse prescribers and that they should use it within the limits of their skills, knowledge and competence (as is the case with dentists who have the BNF at their disposal but only prescribe according to their field of practice).

Latest information from the Department of Health website suggests that from Spring 2006, qualified Extended Formulary Nurse Prescribers will be able to prescribe any licensed medicine for any medical condition, with the exception of controlled drugs.[12]

References

1 Department of Health (1968) *Medicines Act 1968*. HMSO, London.
2 Department of Health (1997) *Prescription Only Medicines Order 1997*. HMSO, London.
3 Department of Health (1980) *Medicines Order 1980*. HMSO, London.
4 Department of Health (2003) *Prescription Only Medicines Amendment Order 2003*. HMSO, London.
5 Department of Health (1971) *Misuse of Drugs Act 1971*. HMSO, London.
6 Department of Health (1992) *Medicinal Products Prescription by Nurses Act 1992*. HMSO, London.
7 Department of Health (1977) *NHS Act 1977*. HMSO, London.
8 Department of Health (2001) *Health and Social Care Act 2001*. HMSO, London.
9 Department of Health (1998) *The Review Team of the Prescribing, Supply and Administration of Medicines*. HMSO, London.
10 Department of Health (2000) *Prescription Only Medicines Amendment Order 2000*. HMSO, London.
11 Clinical Effectiveness Unit (2005) The use of contraception outside the terms of the product licence. *Journal of Family Planning and Reproductive Health Care*. **31** (3): 225–42.
12 Department of Health (2005) *Independent Nurse Prescribing*. www.dh.gov.uk/ PolicyAndGuidance/MedicinesPharmacyAndIndustry/Prescriptions/Nonmedical Prescribing/NursePrescribing/fs/en

Useful resources

• Core Prescribing Group (2005) *Medicine Matters: a guide to correct mechanisms for the prescribing, supply and administration of medicines*. NHS Modernisation Agency Changing Workforce Programme. Department of Health, London.
• National electronic Library for Medicines (2004) *Background Information on Using the National PGD Templates*. December. www.nelm.nhs.uk/PGD/View Recordaspx?recordID=4218referer=http://www.nelm.nhs.uk/PGD/pgddoc. aspx
• NHS National Prescribing Centre (2004) *PGDs: a practical guide and framework of competencies for all professionals using patient group directions, March 2004*. A guide to good practice which incorporates a competency framework for using patient group directions. www.npc.co.uk/publications/pgd/pgd.htm

With thanks to King's College London e-learning courses: Prescribing for Nurses and Pharmacists, 2004.

Aciclovir

Legal classification

POM.

Route of administration

Oral.

Pharmacodynamics

Aciclovir is a pharmacologically inactive guanosine analogue that only becomes a virustatic agent after penetrating into a cell infected by herpes simplex virus (HSV) or varicella zoster virus (VZV). The activation of the aciclovir is catalysed by HSV or VZV thymidine kinase, an enzyme that the virus depends on for replication. In simplified terms, the virus synthesises its own virustatic agent.

Indications

Management of herpes simplex, especially genital herpes infections of skin and mucous membranes (first as well as recurrent episodes).

Contraindications

- Hypersensitivity.
- *Ciclosporin*: increased risk of nephrotoxicity when aciclovir given with ciclosporin.
- *Mycophenolate mofetil*: plasma concentration of aciclovir increased by mycophenolate mofetil; also plasma concentration of inactive metabolite of mycophenolate mofetil increased.

Drug interactions

Probenecid has been shown to reduce the renal clearance of aciclovir by approximately 30%, resulting in an increase of its mean elimination half-life.

Side effects

- Cutaneous reactions that usually disappear after cessation of therapy.
- Gastrointestinal disorders such as nausea, vomiting, diarrhoea and abdominal pain.

Pregnancy and lactation

Use in pregnancy

There is little experience of the administration of oral aciclovir during pregnancy. The use of aciclovir in women who are or may become pregnant requires that an expected benefit is weighed against the possible risks, particularly in the first trimester.

Systemic administration (oral and intravenous administration) of aciclovir during the second and third trimester of pregnancy has been described in some cases without any harm to the foetus.

Use in lactation

After oral administration of aciclovir, five times daily, aciclovir concentrations found in breast milk were 0.6–4.1 times the corresponding aciclovir plasma concentrations. The infant would then receive up to 0.3 mg/kg/day. Mothers should stop nursing during treatment with aciclovir tablets.

Ampicillin

Legal classification

POM.

Route of administration

Oral.

Pharmacodynamics

Ampicillin provides broad-spectrum activity.

Indications

Ampicillin is indicated for the treatment of severe infections where the causative organism is unknown, and for mixed infections involving β-lactamase-producing staphylococci.

Contraindications

- Ampicillin is a penicillin and should not be given to patients with a history of hypersensitivity to β-lactam antibiotics (e.g. penicillins, cephalosporins).
- Ampicillin should be used with caution in patients with evidence of hepatic dysfunction.

Drug interactions

- Bacteriostatic drugs may interfere with the bactericidal action of ampicillin.
- In common with other oral broad-spectrum antibiotics, ampicillin may reduce the efficacy of oral contraceptives.
- Probenecid decreases the renal tubular secretion of ampicillin. Concurrent use with ampicillin may result in increased and prolonged blood levels of ampicillin.
- Concurrent administration of allopurinol during treatment with ampicillin can increase the likelihood of allergic skin reaction.

Side effects

Generally well tolerated.

Pregnancy and lactation

Use in pregnancy

Animal studies with ampicillin have shown no teratogenic effects.

Use in lactation

Trace quantities of ampicillin can be detected in breast milk. The possibility of hypersensitivity reactions must be considered in breastfed infants. Therefore ampicillin should only be administered to a breastfeeding mother when the potential benefit outweighs the potential risks associated with treatment.

Azithromycin

Legal classification

POM.

Route of administration

Oral.

Pharmacodynamics

Azithromycin is an azalide, derived from the macrolide class of antibiotics. The mode of action of azithromycin is inhibition of protein synthesis in bacteria by binding to the 50s ribosomal subunit and preventing translocation of peptides.

Indications

- Azithromycin is indicated in the treatment of uncomplicated genital infections due to *Chlamydia trachomatis.*
- Azithromycin should be given as a single daily dose. In common with many other antibiotics, azithromycin should be taken at least one hour before or two hours after food.

Contraindications

- Known hypersensitivity.
- *Use in renal impairment:* In patients with severe renal impairment (GFR <10 ml/min) a 33% increase in systemic exposure to azithromycin was observed.
- *Use in hepatic impairment:* As the liver is the principal route of excretion of azithromycin, it should not be used in patients with hepatic disease.

Drug interactions

- *Antacids:* In patients receiving azithromycin and antacids, azithromycin should be taken at least one hour before or two hours after the antacid.
- *Cyclosporin:* In a pharmacokinetic study with healthy volunteers that were administered a 500 mg/day oral dose of azithromycin for three days and were then administered a single 10 mg/kg oral dose of cyclosporin, the resulting cyclosporin was found to be significantly elevated. Consequently, caution should be exercised before considering co-administration of these two drugs. If co-administration is necessary, cyclosporin levels should be monitored and the dose adjusted accordingly.
- *Digoxin:* Some of the macrolide antibiotics have been reported to impair the metabolism of digoxin (in the gut) in some patients. Therefore, in patients receiving concomitant azithromycin and digoxin the possibility of raised digoxin levels should be borne in mind, and digoxin levels monitored.
- *Ergot derivatives:* Because of the theoretical possibility of ergotism, azithromycin and ergot derivatives should not be co-administered.
- *Theophylline:* Theophylline levels may be increased in patients taking azithromycin.

Side effects

Azithromycin is well tolerated with a low incidence of side effects.

Pregnancy and lactation

Use in pregnancy

Animal reproduction studies have demonstrated that azithromycin crosses the placenta, but have revealed no evidence of harm to the foetus. There are no adequate and well-controlled studies in pregnant women. Since animal studies are not always predictive of human response, azithromycin should be used during pregnancy only if adequate alternatives are not available.

Use in lactation

No data on secretion of azithromycin in breast milk are available, so azithromycin should only be used in lactating women where adequate alternatives are not available.

Cefixime

Legal classification

POM.

Route of administration

Oral.

Pharmacodynamics

Cefixime is an orally active cephalosporin antibiotic which has marked *in vitro* bactericidal activity against a wide variety of Gram-positive and Gram-negative organisms.

Indications

Gonorrhoea.

Contraindications

- Patients with known hypersensitivity to cephalosporin antibiotics.
- Cephalosporins should be given with caution to penicillin-sensitive patients, as there is some evidence of partial cross-allergenicity between the penicillins and cephalosporins.

Drug interactions

In common with other cephalosporins, increases in prothrombin times have been noted in a few patients. Care should therefore be taken in patients receiving anticoagulation therapy.

Side effects

Mild and self-limiting in nature.

Pregnancy and lactation

There are no adequate and well-controlled studies in pregnant women. Cefixime should therefore not be used in pregnancy or in nursing mothers unless considered essential.

Ceftriaxone

Legal classification

POM.

Route of administration

IM/IV.

Pharmacodynamics

Ceftriaxone has potent bactericidal activity against a wide range of Gram-positive and, especially, Gram-negative organisms. The spectrum of activity includes both aerobic and some anaerobic species. It has considerable resistance to degradation by most bacterial β-lactamases.

Indications

Ceftriaxone sodium is a broad-spectrum bactericidal cephalosporin antibiotic. Ceftriaxone is active *in vitro* against a wide range of Gram-positive and Gram-negative organisms, which include β-lactamase-producing strains.

Contraindications

- In patients with liver damage there is no need for the dosage to be reduced provided renal function is intact.
- In severe renal impairment accompanied by hepatic insufficiency, the plasma concentration of ceftriaxone should be determined at regular intervals and dosage adjusted.
- In patients undergoing dialysis, no additional supplementary dosage is required following the dialysis. Plasma concentrations should be monitored, however, to determine whether dosage adjustments are necessary, since the elimination rate in these patients may be reduced.
- Care is required when administering ceftriaxone to patients who have previously shown hypersensitivity (especially anaphylactic reaction) to penicillins or other non-cephalosporin β-lactam antibiotics, as occasional instances of cross-allergenicity between cephalosporins and these antibiotics have been recorded.

Drug interactions

- In an *in vitro* study, antagonistic effects have been observed with the combination of chloramphenicol and ceftriaxone.
- Ceftriaxone is not compatible with calcium-containing solutions such as Hartmann's solution and Ringer's solution.
- Based on literature reports, ceftriaxone is not compatible with amsacrine, vancomycin, fluconazole, aminoglycosides and labetalol.

Side effects

- Ceftriaxone may precipitate in the gall bladder and then be detectable as shadows on ultrasound. This can happen in patients of any age, but is more likely in infants and small children who are usually given a larger dose of ceftriaxone on a body-weight basis.
- Ceftriaxone has been generally well tolerated. Adverse reactions are usually mild and transient.
- The most common side effects are gastrointestinal, consisting mainly of loose stools and diarrhoea, nausea and vomiting, stomatitis and glossitis.
- Superinfections with yeasts, fungi or other resistant organisms may occur.

- Pain or discomfort may be experienced at the site of intramuscular injection immediately after administration but is usually well tolerated and transient. Local phlebitis has occurred rarely following intravenous administration but can be minimised by slow injection over at least 2–4 minutes.

Pregnancy and lactation

Use in pregnancy

Ceftriaxone has not been associated with adverse events on foetal development in laboratory animals but its safety in human pregnancy has not been established; therefore it should not be used in pregnancy unless absolutely indicated.

Use in lactation

Only minimal amounts of ceftriaxone are excreted in breast milk. However, caution is advised in nursing mothers.

Ciprofloxacin

Legal classification

POM.

Route of administration

Oral.

Pharmacodynamics

Ciprofloxacin is a synthetic 4-quinolone derivative, with bactericidal activity. It acts via inhibition of bacterial DNA gyrase, ultimately resulting in interference with DNA function. Ciprofloxacin is highly active against a wide range of Gram-positive and Gram-negative organisms and has shown activity against some anaerobes.

Indications

- PID.
- Chancroid.
- Gonorrhoea.

Contraindications

- Ciprofloxacin is contraindicated in patients who have shown hypersensitivity to ciprofloxacin or other quinolone anti-infectives.

- Ciprofloxacin is contraindicated in children and growing adolescents unless the benefits of treatment are considered to outweigh the risks.
- Ciprofloxacin should be used with caution in epileptics and patients with a history of central nervous system (CNS) disorders and only if the benefits of treatment are considered to outweigh the risk of possible CNS side effects. CNS side effects have been reported after first administration of ciprofloxacin in some patients. Treatment should be discontinued if the side effects, depression or psychoses lead to self-endangering behaviour.

Drug interactions

- Ciprofloxacin tablets should not be administered within four hours of multivalent cationic drugs and mineral supplements (e.g. calcium, magnesium, aluminium or iron), sucralfate or antacids and highly buffered drugs (e.g. didanosine) as interference with absorption may occur. When appropriate, patients should be advised not to self-medicate with preparations containing these compounds during therapy with ciprofloxacin.
- Increased plasma levels of theophylline have been observed following concurrent administration with ciprofloxacin. It is recommended that the dose of theophylline should be reduced and plasma levels of theophylline monitored. The reaction between theophylline and ciprofloxacin is potentially life-threatening. Therefore, where monitoring of plasma levels is not possible, the use of ciprofloxacin should be avoided in patients receiving theophylline. Particular caution is advised in those patients with convulsive disorders.
- Phenytoin levels may be altered when ciprofloxacin is used concomitantly.
- Renal tubular transport of methotrexate may be inhibited by concomitant administration of ciprofloxacin, potentially leading to increased plasma levels of methotrexate. This may increase the risk of methotrexate-associated toxic reactions. Therefore, patients receiving methotrexate therapy should be carefully monitored when concomitant ciprofloxacin therapy is indicated.
- Concomitant use with probenecid reduces the renal clearance of ciprofloxacin, resulting in increased quinolone plasma levels.
- Animal data have shown that high doses of quinolones, in combination with some non-steroidal anti-inflammatory drugs, can lead to convulsions.
- The use of metoclopramide with ciprofloxacin may accelerate the absorption of ciprofloxacin.

Side effects

- Crystalluria related to the use of ciprofloxacin has been reported. Patients receiving ciprofloxacin should be well hydrated and excessive alkalinity of the urine should be avoided.
- Patients with a family history of or actual defects in glucose-6-phosphate dehydrogenase activity are prone to haemolytic reactions with quinolones, and so ciprofloxacin should be used with caution in these patients.
- As with other quinolones, patients should avoid prolonged exposure to strong sunlight or ultraviolet (UV) radiation during treatment.
- Ciprofloxacin could result in impairment of the patient's ability to drive or operate machinery, particularly in conjunction with alcohol.

- Ciprofloxacin is generally well tolerated. The most frequently reported adverse reactions are nausea, diarrhoea and rash.

Pregnancy and lactation

Use in pregnancy

As with other quinolones, ciprofloxacin has been shown to cause arthropathy in immature animals, and therefore its use during pregnancy is not recommended.

Use in lactation

Studies have indicated that ciprofloxacin is secreted in breast milk. Administration to nursing mothers is thus not recommended.

Clotrimazole

Legal classification

P.

Route of administration

PV/topical.

Pharmacodynamics

The antimycotic effect of clotrimazole is primarily fungistatic, and at high concentrations also fungicidal. Clotrimazole is only effective against proliferating fungi. Current knowledge indicates that the antimycotic effect of clotrimazole is due to inhibition of ergosterin biosynthesis. Ergosterin is an essential component of the fungal cell membrane. Under the influence of clotrimazole, its biosynthesis is delayed – with this being due to the consumption of cytoplasmic ergosterin in the fungal cell. Severe changes in the composition and properties of the membrane result, and these changes are then linked to the disturbed membrane permeability, leading finally to cytolysis.

In addition, at fungistatic concentrations, clotrimazole interferes with mitochondrial and peroxisomal enzymes. A toxic increase in the hydrogen peroxide concentration results, probably contributing to cell death (hydrogen peroxide autodigestion).

Indications

Candidal vaginitis.

Contraindications

Clotrimazole should not be administered in cases of hypersensitivity to clotrimazole or any of the other ingredients.

Drug interactions

Clotrimazole reduces the efficacy of other drugs which are used for the treatment of fungal diseases (amphotericin and other polyene antibiotics, e.g. nystatin).

Side effects

Rarely, patients may experience local mild burning or irritation immediately after applying the vaginal tablet. Very rarely the patient may find this irritation intolerable and stop treatment. Hypersensitivity reactions may occur.

Pregnancy and lactation

Use in pregnancy

In animal studies clotrimazole has not been associated with teratogenic effects, but following oral administration of high doses to rats there was evidence of foetotoxicity. The relevance of this effect to topical application in humans is not known. However, clotrimazole has been used in pregnant patients for over a decade without adverse effects. It is therefore recommended that clotrimazole should be used in pregnancy only when considered necessary by the health professional.

As a measure of precaution clotrimazole vaginal tablets should not be used in early pregnancy.

Use in lactation

Clotrimazole can be used during lactation.

Condyline™

See Podophyllotoxin.

Cryotherapy

Legal classification

POM.

Route of administration

Topical.

Pharmacodynamics

There is no specific antiviral therapy against the human papilloma virus. Treatment usually relies on some form of local tissue destruction. Solid carbon dioxide, or 'dry ice', has a temperature of minus 80 degrees and has been used to treat warts, molluscum and naevi by cryotherapy.

Indications

- Warts.
- Molluscum.

Contraindications

Nil.

Drug interactions

There are no known drug interactions with cryotherapy.

Side effects

- Mild to moderate burning sensation during the procedure. Irritation, soreness, or mild pain may occur after the procedure.
- Swelling.
- Shedding of dead tissue.
- Sores or blisters may form.

Pregnancy and lactation

Cryotherapy can be used in pregnancy and during lactation.

Doxycycline

Legal classification

POM.

Route of administration

Oral.

Pharmacodynamics

Doxycycline is clinically effective in the treatment of a variety of infections caused by sensitive strains of Gram-negative and Gram-positive bacteria, as well as certain other micro-organisms. As an antibiotic, doxycycline exerts its anti-microbial effect by the inhibition of protein synthesis and is considered to be primarily bacteriostatic.

Indications

- NGU.
- Chlamydia.
- Syphilis.

Contraindications

- Hypersensitivity to doxycycline, any of the capsule excipients or to any of the tetracyclines.
- Systemic lupus erythematosus.
- Porphyria.
- Achlorhydria.
- Impaired hepatic function.
- Impaired renal function.

Drug interactions

- Concurrent administration of medicaments containing the following may impair the absorption of doxycycline: antacids containing magnesium, aluminium or calcium salts; oral zinc, iron salts or bismuth preparations.
- Since bacteriostatic drugs may interfere with the bactericidal action of penicillin, it is advisable to avoid giving doxycycline in conjunction with penicillin.
- Since tetracyclines depress plasma prothrombin activity, reduced dosages of concomitant anti-coagulants may be required.
- Concurrent administration of barbiturates, carbamazepine or phenytoin may decrease the serum half-life of doxycycline, and may necessitate an increase in the daily dosage of doxycycline.
- The concurrent use of tetracyclines and methoxyflurane has been reported to result in fatal renal toxicity.
- Alcohol may decrease the half-life of doxycycline.
- Doxycycline may possibly increase plasma-cyclosporin concentrations, on concomitant administration.
- There is a chance of an increased risk of benign intracranial hypertension with the administration of tetracyclines with the retinoids acitretin, isotretinoin or tretinoin.
- Tetracyclines may increase plasma concentrations of digoxin or lithium.
- Care should be taken with the concomitant administration of tetracyclines with diuretics, since there may be an exacerbation of possible nephrotoxicity.
- A few cases of pregnancy or breakthrough bleeding have been attributed to the concurrent use of tetracycline antibiotics with oral contraceptives.
- Care should be taken with the concomitant use of doxycycline with other drugs which can inhibit or induce hepatic metabolism or with drugs which are potentially hepatotoxic.

Side effects

- Doxycycline can cause oesophageal irritation and ulceration when taken orally. Administration of doxycycline capsules with adequate amounts of fluid is therefore recommended, well before retiring at night, to reduce this risk.
- The use of tetracycline drugs (which include doxycycline) during tooth development (pregnancy, infancy and childhood up to 12 years old) may cause permanent discolouration of the teeth (yellow–grey–brown). This adverse

effect is more common during long-term therapy but has been observed following repeated short-term courses.

- Tetracyclines have been reported to cause photosensitivity, apparently as an exaggerated reaction to sunlight, and allergic skin reactions in some patients taking doxycycline. Patients should be advised to avoid exposure to direct sunlight or ultraviolet light and told that treatment should be discontinued at the first signs of skin discomfort or erythema.
- Microbiological overgrowth: the use of antibiotics may occasionally result in overgrowth of non-susceptible organisms including *Candida albicans*. If a resistant organism appears, the antibiotic should be discontinued and appropriate therapy instituted.

Pregnancy and lactation

Use in pregnancy

Doxycycline is contraindicated in pregnancy and in breastfeeding mothers. Results of animal studies indicate that tetracyclines cross the placenta, are found in foetal tissues and can have toxic effects on the developing foetus (often related to retardation of skeletal development). Evidence of embryotoxicity has also been noted in animals treated early in pregnancy.

Use in lactation

Tetracyclines are excreted in breast milk and are therefore contraindicated in nursing mothers (*see* above reference to use during tooth development).

Erythromycin

Legal classification

POM.

Route of administration

Oral.

Pharmacodynamics

Erythromycin exerts its antimicrobial action by binding to the 50S ribosomal subunit of susceptible micro-organisms and suppresses protein synthesis.

Indications

- Chlamydia.
- PID.
- Syphilis.

Contraindications

- Known hypersensitivity.
- Erythromycin is excreted principally by the liver, so caution should be exercised in administering the antibiotic to patients with impaired hepatic function or concomitantly receiving potentially hepatotoxic agents.

Drug interactions

Alfentanil	Disopyramide	Theophylline
Astemizole	Ergotamine	Triazolam
Bromocriptine	Hexobarbitone	Valproate
Carbamazapine	Midazolam	Warfarin
Cisapride	Phenytoin	
Clarithromycin	Pimozide	
Cyclosporin	Guinidine	
Digoxin	Tacrolimus	
Dihydroergotamine	Terfenadine	

- Concomitant use of erythromycin with terfenadine or astemizole is likely to result in an enhanced risk of cardiotoxicity with these drugs. The metabolism of terfenadine and astemizole is significantly altered when either are taken concomitantly with erythromycin. Rare cases of serious cardiovascular events have been observed, including torsades de pointes, other ventricular arrhythmias and cardiac arrest. Death has been reported with the terfenadine/erythromycin combination.
- Elevated cisapride levels have been reported in patients receiving erythromycin and cisapride concomitantly. This may result in QT prolongation and cardiac arrhythmias, including ventricular tachycardia, ventricular fibrillation and torsades de pointes.
- Similar effects have been observed with concomitant administration of pimozide and clarithromycin, another macrolide antibiotic.
- Concurrent use of erythromycin and ergotamine or dihydroergotamine has been associated in some patients with acute ergot toxicity characterised by the rapid development of severe peripheral vasospasm and dysaesthesia.
- Increases in serum concentrations of the following drugs metabolised by the cytochrome P450 system may occur when administered concurrently with erythromycin: alfentanil, astemizole, bromocriptine, carbamazepine, cyclosporin, digoxin, dihydroergotamine, disopyramide, ergotamine, hexobarbitone, midazolam, phenytoin, quinidine, tacrolimus, terfenadine, theophylline, triazolam, valproate and warfarin. Appropriate monitoring should be undertaken and dosage should be adjusted as necessary.
- Erythromycin has been reported to decrease the clearance of zopiclone and thus may increase the pharmacodynamic effects of this drug.
- When oral erythromycin is given concurrently with theophylline, there is a significant decrease in erythromycin serum concentrations. The decrease could result in subtherapeutic concentrations of erythromycin.

Side effects

Few and transient.

Pregnancy and lactation

Use in pregnancy

There is no evidence of hazard from erythromycin in human pregnancy. It has been in widespread use for a number of years without apparent ill consequence.

Use in lactation

Erythromycin is excreted in breast milk, therefore caution should be exercised when erythromycin is administered to a nursing mother.

Hepatitis A vaccine

Legal classification

POM.

Route of administration

IM.

Pharmacodynamics

Active immunisation against hepatitis A virus (HAV). In haemodialysis patients and in subjects with an impaired immune system, adequate anti-HAV antibody titres may not be obtained after the primary immunisation and such patients may therefore require administration of additional doses of vaccine.

Indications

Active immunisation against infections caused by hepatitis A virus. The vaccine is particularly indicated for those at increased risk of infection or transmission. For example, immunisation should be considered for the following risk groups:

- travellers visiting areas of medium or high endemicity, i.e. anywhere outside northern or western Europe, Australia, North America and New Zealand
- military and diplomatic personnel, haemophiliacs and patients, intravenous drug abusers, homosexual men, laboratory workers working directly with the hepatitis A virus, sanitation workers in contact with untreated sewage
- patients with chronic liver disease (including alcoholic cirrhosis, chronic hepatitis B, chronic hepatitis C, autoimmune hepatitis, primary biliary cirrhosis)
- close contacts of hepatitis A cases
- since virus shedding from infected persons may occur for a prolonged period, active immunisation of close contacts may be considered.

Contraindications

- Hypersensitivity to any vaccine component or hypersensitivity following a previous injection of this vaccine.
- Systemic hypersensitivity to neomycin, which may be present in the vaccine in trace amounts.
- Vaccination should be delayed in subjects with an acute severe febrile illness.

Drug interactions

Preliminary data on the concomitant administration of hepatitis A vaccine with recombinant hepatitis B virus vaccine suggest that there is no interference in the immune response to either antigen. On this basis and since it is an inactivated vaccine, interference with immune response is unlikely to occur when hepatitis A vaccine is administered with other inactivated or live vaccines. When concomitant administration is considered necessary the vaccines must be given at different injection sites. Hepatitis A vaccine must not be mixed with other vaccines in the same syringe.

Side effects

- These are usually mild and confined to the first few days after vaccination. The most common reactions are mild transient soreness, erythema and induration at the injection site.
- Less common general complaints, not necessarily related to the vaccination, include headache, fever, malaise, fatigue, nausea, diarrhoea, loss of appetite and rash.
- Arthralgia, myalgia, convulsions and allergic reactions including anaphylactoid reactions have been reported very rarely.
- Elevations of serum liver enzymes (usually transient) have been reported occasionally. However, a causal relationship with the vaccine has not been established.

Pregnancy and lactation

Use in pregnancy

The effect of hepatitis A vaccine on foetal development has not been assessed. However, as with all inactivated viral vaccines, the risks to the foetus are considered negligible. Hepatitis A vaccine should be used during pregnancy only when clearly needed.

Use in lactation

The effect on breastfed infants of the administration of hepatitis A vaccine to their mothers has not been evaluated in clinical studies. Hepatitis A vaccine should therefore be used with caution in breastfeeding women.

Hepatitis B vaccine

Legal classification

POM.

Route of administration

IM. The immune response to hepatitis B vaccine is affected by the site of intramuscular injection. The deltoid region is recommended for adults and the anterolateral thigh for infants. A diminished response has been associated with administration in the gluteal region (buttock).

Pharmacodynamics

Active immunisation against hepatitis B virus.

Indications

The World Health Organization recommended that national immunisation policies should include routine hepatitis B immunisation for the whole population by 1997 and this has been implemented in some countries. The current recommendations in the UK are for immunisation of persons at high risk of contracting hepatitis B. High-risk groups include:

- healthcare personnel
- laboratory workers, or any other personnel who have direct contact with patients or their body fluids or tissues
- staff and residents of accommodation for those with severe learning difficulties
- patients with chronic renal failure, including those requiring haemodialysis, haemophiliacs and those receiving regular blood transfusions or blood products
- close family contacts or sexual partners of cases or carriers of hepatitis B
- families adopting children from countries with a high prevalence of hepatitis B
- individuals who frequently change sexual partners
- parenteral drug abusers
- inmates of custodial institutions
- some travellers to areas where hepatitis B is endemic
- immunisation should also be performed in infants born to women who are persistent carriers of hepatitis B surface antigen or infants born to women who are HBsAg-positive as a result of recent infection
- hepatitis C carriers who are not immunised against hepatitis B should also receive immunisation.

Contraindications

- Hypersensitivity to any component of the vaccine.
- Acute febrile illness.

- Some studies have observed a defective response in chronic alcoholics whereas others have not; the degree of liver impairment may be a significant factor. It has been suggested that an increased dose of hepatitis B vaccine may be appropriate in those with a history of alcoholism. A diminished response occurs in HIV-positive patients.
- In patients on haemodialysis; an increased dose of hepatitis B vaccine is recommended in these patients.
- In patients with haemophilia who are not HIV-positive.

Drug interactions

No known drug interactions.

Side effects

No serious adverse reactions attributable to the vaccine have been reported during the course of clinical trials.

- Injection of a vaccine may be followed by a local reaction, possibly with inflammation and lymphangitis. An induration or sterile abscess may develop at the site of injected vaccine.
- Fever, headache and malaise may start a few hours after injection and last for one or two days.
- Hypersensitivity reactions may occur and anaphylaxis has been reported rarely.
- In addition, hepatitis B vaccines have been reported to cause abdominal pain and gastrointestinal disturbance, and musculoskeletal and joint pain and inflammation. There may also be dizziness and sleep disturbance. Cardiovascular effects include occasional hypotension and, rarely, tachycardia. Other rare adverse effects include dysuria, visual disturbances and earache.

Pregnancy and lactation

Use in pregnancy

The effect of the HBsAg on foetal development has not been assessed. However, as with all inactivated viral vaccines, one does not expect harm for the foetus. Hepatitis B vaccine should be used during pregnancy only when clearly needed, and the possible advantages outweigh the possible risks for the foetus.

Use in lactation

The effect on breastfed infants of the administration of hepatitis B vaccine to their mothers has not been evaluated in clinical studies, as information concerning the excretion into the breast milk is not available. No contraindication has been established.

Imiquimod cream

Legal classification

POM.

Route of administration

Topical.

Pharmacodynamics

Imiquimod is an immune-response modifier. Saturable binding studies suggest a membrane receptor for imiquimod exists on responding immune cells. Imiquimod has no direct antiviral activity. In animal models imiquimod is effective against viral infections and acts as an antitumour agent principally by induction of alpha interferon and other cytokines. The induction of alpha interferon and other cytokines following imiquimod cream application to genital wart tissue has also been demonstrated in clinical studies.

Indications

- HPV.
- Anogenital warts.
- Molluscum.

Contraindications

- Imiquimod cream is contraindicated in patients with known hypersensitivity to imiquimod or any of the excipients of the cream.
- In immunocompromised patients, repeat treatment with imiquimod cream is not recommended.

Drug interactions

Interactions with other medicinal products, including immunosuppressive drugs, have not been studied; such interactions with systemic drugs would be limited by the minimal percutaneous absorption of imiquimod cream.

Side effects

Local skin reactions such as erythema, erosion, excoriation, flaking and oedema are common. Other local reactions such as induration, ulceration, scabbing and vesicles have also been reported. Should an intolerable skin reaction occur, the cream should be removed by washing the area with mild soap and water. Treatment with imiquimod cream can be resumed after the skin reaction has moderated.

Pregnancy and lactation

Use in pregnancy

In animal teratology and reproductive studies, no teratogenic nor embryo-foetotoxic effects were observed. In the absence of such effects in animals, malformative effects in man are generally considered unlikely to occur. However, caution should be exercised when prescribing to pregnant women.

Use in lactation

As no quantifiable levels of imiquimod are detected in the serum after single and multiple topical doses, no specific advice can be given on whether to use or not in lactating mothers.

Malathion

Legal classification

POM.

Route of administration

Topical.

Pharmacodynamics

Malathion is a widely used organophosphorus insecticide which is active by cholinesterase inhibition. It is effective against a wide range of insects, but is one of the least toxic organophosphorus insecticides since it is rapidly detoxified by plasma carboxylesterases.

Indications

- Pubic lice.
- Scabies.

Contraindications

- Known sensitivity to malathion.
- Not to be used on infants less than six months except on medical advice.

Drug interactions

Nil known.

Side effects

Some local reactions may occur.

Pregnancy and lactation

No known effects in pregnancy and lactation. However, as with all medicines, use with caution.

Metronidazole

Legal classification

POM.

Route of administration

Oral/PV.

Pharmacodynamics

Metronidazole is a synthetic antibacterial agent which also possesses amoebicidal activity.

Indications

- Bacterial vaginosis.
- PID.
- Trichomonas.

Contraindications

- Patients with a prior history of hypersensitivity to metronidazole, other nitroimidazoles, or parabens.
- Metronidazole is a nitroimidazole and should be used with care in patients with evidence of a history of blood dyscrasias.
- As with all vaginal infections, sexual intercourse during the infection and during treatment with metronidazole vaginal gel is not recommended.

Drug interactions

Oral metronidazole has been shown to increase the plasma concentrations of warfarin, lithium, cyclosporin and 5-fluorouracil. Similar effects after vaginal administration of metronidazole are not expected due to the low plasma concentrations but cannot be completely ruled out.

Side effects

- Known or previously unrecognised candidiasis may present more prominent symptoms during therapy with vaginal gel and may require treatment with a candicidal agent.

- Oral metronidazole has been associated with a disulfiram-like reaction in combination with alcohol. At the low serum concentrations which result from the use of metronidazole vaginal gel, the possibility of similar reactions is unlikely although cannot be excluded.
- The most commonly reported adverse drug reactions were urogenital and gastrointestinal.

Pregnancy and lactation

Use in pregnancy

Data on a large number of exposed pregnancies indicate no adverse effects of metronidazole on the foetus/newborn child.

Use in lactation

Metronidazole is excreted in milk at concentrations similar to those in maternal serum; caution should be exercised when prescribing to lactating women.

Miconazole

Legal classification

POM.

Route of administration

PV.

Pharmacodynamics

Miconazole is a synthetic imidazole antifungal agent with a broad spectrum of activity against pathogenic fungi (including yeasts and dermatophytes) and Gram-positive bacteria. There is little absorption through mucous membranes when miconazole is applied topically.

Indications

Candida.

Contraindications

Nil known.

Drug interactions

Contact should be avoided between contraceptive diaphragms or condoms and miconazole pessaries since they may be damaged by the emollient base.

Side effects

Occasionally, irritation has been reported. Rarely, local sensitisation may occur requiring discontinuation of treatment.

Pregnancy and lactation

In animals, miconazole nitrate has shown no teratogenic effects but is foetotoxic at high oral doses. The significance of this to man is unknown as there is no evidence of increased risk when taken in human pregnancy. However, as with other imidazoles, miconazole should be used in pregnant women only if the practitioner considers it to be necessary.

Nystatin

Legal classification

POM.

Route of administration

PV/topical.

Pharmacodynamics

Nystatin is an antifungal antibiotic active against a wide range of yeasts and yeast-like fungi, including *Candida albicans*. Nystatin is formulated in oral and topical dosage forms and is not systemically absorbed from any of these preparations.

Indications

Candida.

Contraindications

There are no known contraindications to the use of nystatin.

Drug interactions

Avoid contact between the cream and contraceptive diaphragms, caps and condoms, since they may be damaged by the preparation.

Side effects

Some transient local discomfort may be experienced.

Pregnancy and lactation

Use in pregnancy

There is no evidence that nystatin is absorbed systemically from the vagina. However, as with all drugs, caution should be exercised in pregnancy. Care should be taken while using an applicator to prevent the possibility of mechanical trauma.

Use in lactation

Nystatin can be used during lactation.

Permethrin

Legal classification

P.

Route of administration

Topical.

Pharmacodynamics

Permethrin is rapidly absorbed across the insect cuticle. The principal physiological action is the induction of electrochemical abnormalities across the membranes of excitable cells, leading to sensory hyperexcitability, incoordination and prostration. When presented in aqueous base, the ovicidal activity of permethrin is increased by the addition of an alcohol.

Indications

- Public lice.
- Scabies.

Contraindications

Contraindicated in individuals with known hypersensitivity to the product, its components and other pyrethroids or pyrethrins.

Drug interactions

None known.

Side effects

Generally well tolerated with a low potential for inducing skin reactions. In a few individuals, erythema, rash and/or irritation of the scalp have been reported following the application of the creme rinse, but as an infestation with lice is often associated with skin irritation, it is difficult in most instances to determine the underlying cause.

Pregnancy and lactation

Use in pregnancy

Reproduction studies have been performed on animals and have revealed no evidence of impaired fertility or harm to the foetus due to permethrin. There are, however, only very limited data on the use of permethrin in pregnant women. Because animal studies are not always predictive of the human response, treatment should be considered during pregnancy only if clearly needed.

Use in lactation

Studies following oral administration of permethrin in cattle have indicated that very low concentrations of permethrin are excreted in milk. However, it is not known whether permethrin is excreted in human milk. While it is unlikely that the concentrations of permethrin in the milk will present any risk to the infant, consideration should be given to withholding treatment during nursing or temporarily discontinuing nursing.

Podophyllotoxin

Legal classification

POM.

Route of administration

Topical.

Pharmacodynamics

Podophyllotoxin is a metaphase inhibitor in dividing cells binding to at least one binding site on tubulin. Binding prevents tubulin polymerisation required for microtubule assembly. At higher concentrations, podophyllotoxin also inhibits nucleoside transport through the cell membrane.

The chemotherapeutic action of podophyllotoxin is assumed to be due to inhibition of growth and the ability to invade the tissue of the viral infected cells.

Indications

- HPV.
- Anogenital warts.

Contraindications

- Open wounds, e.g. following surgical procedures.
- Use in children.
- Hypersensitivity to podophyllotoxin.
- Concomitant use with other podophyllotoxin-containing preparations.

Drug interactions

Nil known.

Side effects

- The hands should be thoroughly washed after each application. Prolonged contact with healthy skin must be avoided since the cream contains an active pharmaceutical substance which could be harmful on healthy skin.
- Local irritation may occur on the second or third day of application associated with the start of wart necrosis. In most cases the reactions are mild.
- Tenderness, itching, smarting, erythema, superficial epithelial ulceration and balanoposthitis have been reported. Local irritation decreases after treatment.

Pregnancy and lactation

Use in pregnancy

Reproduction toxicity studies in animals have not given evidence of an increased incidence of foetal damage or other deleterious effects on the reproductive process. However, since podophyllotoxin is a mitosis inhibitor, it should not be used during pregnancy.

Use in lactation

It is not known if the substance is excreted into breast milk. Therefore it is recommended that it not be used during lactation.

Probenecid

Legal classification

POM.

Route of administration

Oral.

Pharmacodynamics

Probenecid acts as an active tubular secretion inhibitor and prevents the concomitant drug from being excreted.

Probenecid works on the kidneys to increase the rate at which uric acid is excreted. In gout, crystals of uric acid form in the joints and cause the characteristic pain and inflammation. By lowering the levels of uric acid, gout can be prevented. Although probenecid increases the rate of removal of uric acid in the urine, it actually decreases the rate of removal of certain other medicines, e.g. some antibiotics. This effect has been used to increase the levels of some antibiotics in the body. For example, probenecid is used along with penicillin antibiotics to increase antibiotic blood levels. This increase makes the antibiotic more effective in treating certain infections.

Indications

- Gonorrhoea.
- PID.
- Syphilis.

Contraindications

- History of blood disorders.
- Nephrolithiasis.
- Porphyria.
- Acute gout attack.
- Kidney stones.
- Known sensitivity or allergy to any ingredient.

Drug interactions

- Probenecid increases plasma concentrations of methotrexate in both animals and humans.
- Aspirin and salicylates antagonise the uricosuric action of probenecid.
- Alcohol may worsen the condition.

Side effects

- Nausea.
- Loss of appetite.
- Drowsiness.
- Vomiting.
- Headache.
- Sore gums.
- Frequent urination.

Pregnancy and lactation

Use in pregnancy

This medicine should be used with caution during pregnancy, and only if the expected benefit to the mother is greater than the possible risk to the foetus.

Use in lactation

This medicine should be used with caution by breastfeeding mothers, and only if the expected benefit to the mother is greater than the possible risk to the foetus.

Spectinomycin

Legal classification

POM.

Route of administration

IM.

Pharmacodynamics

Spectinomycin is an aminocyclitol antibacterial that acts by binding to the 30S subunit of the bacterial ribosome and inhibiting protein synthesis. Its activity is generally modest, particularly against Gram-positive organisms. Anaerobic organisms are mostly resistant. Although generally bacteriostatic, spectinomycin is bactericidal against susceptible gonococci.

Indications

Gonorrhoea (spectinomycin will not work for gonorrhoea of the throat).

Contraindications

Sensitivity to drug and any of its incipients.

Drug interactions

Lithium toxicity has been reported on isolated occasions.

Side effects

- Soreness at the injection site.
- Urticaria.
- Dizziness.
- Nausea.
- Chills.
- Fever.
- Insomnia.

Pregnancy and lactation

Use in pregnancy

Studies have not been done in humans. However, spectinomycin has been recommended for the treatment of gonorrhoea and related infections in pregnant patients who are allergic to penicillins, cephalosporins, or probenecid. In addition, studies in animals have not shown that spectinomycin causes birth defects or other problems.

Use in lactation

It is not known if spectinomycin passes into breast milk. However, spectinomycin has not been reported to cause problems in nursing babies.

Trichloracetic acid

See Podophyllotoxin.

Valaciclovir

See aciclovir.

Warticon^{TM}

See Podophyllotoxin.

Glossary

Ablative – taking away or removing.

Achlorhydria – the absence of hydrochloric acid from the gastric juice.

Actinomyces – a genus of Gram-positive, rod-shaped bacteria whose organisms are non-motile.

ALT (alanine transaminase) – a liver enzyme that plays a role in protein metabolism, like AST. Elevated serum levels of ALT are a sign of liver damage from disease or drugs. Synonym: serum glutamic pyruvic transaminase.

Aminoglycosides – a group of antibiotics active against many aerobic Gram-negative and some Gram-positive bacteria. They are mostly produced by fungi and contain an amino sugar, and amino- or guanido-substituted inositol ring; these are attached by a glycosidic linkage to a hexose nucleus, resulting in a polycationic and highly polar compound. They inhibit bacterial protein synthesis by binding to a site on the 30S ribosomal subunit, thereby altering codon and anticodon recognition. They are all broad-spectrum antibiotics and can cause renal toxicity and ototoxicity. Common examples are streptomycin, gentamicin, amikacin, kanamycin, tobramycin, netilmicin, neomycin, framycetin.

Amsell criteria – in clinical practice bacterial vaginosis (BV) is diagnosed using the Amsel criteria (Amsel *et al.* 1983).[1] At least three of the four criteria are present for the diagnosis to be confirmed:

1 thin, white, homogeneous discharge
2 clue cells on microscopy
3 pH of vaginal fluid >4.5
4 release of a fishy odour on adding alkali (10% KOH).

Antimetemolite – a drug that is similar enough to a natural chemical to participate in a normal biochemical reaction in cells but different enough to interfere with the normal division and functions of cells. So named because the drug inhibits a normal metabolic process.

Antimycotic – suppressing the growth of fungi.

Aphasia – loss or impairment of the power to use or comprehend words, usually resulting from brain damage.

Arthralgia – pain in a joint.

AST (aspartate transaminase) – an enzyme present in hepatocytes and myocytes that catalyses the reversible transfer of an amine group from l-glutamic acid to oxaloacetic acid, forming alpha-ketoglutaric acid and l-aspartic acid. It is raised in conditions that affect the heart and liver such as viral hepatitis and myocardial infarction. Following damage to these cells, the enzyme is released into the blood where the level can be measured. Synonym: glutamic-aspartic transaminase, glutamic-oxaloacetic transaminase, serum glutamic-oxaloacetic transaminase.

Azole – a heterocyclic compound found in many biologically important substances.

Balanoposthitis – inflammation of the glans penis and prepuce is often caused by a bacterial infection with *Staphylococcus aureus*.

Behçet's disease – a multisystem, chronic recurrent disease characterised by ulceration in the mouth and genitalia, iritis, uveitis, arthritis and thrombophlebitis.

Carbarnate – pesticide.

Catatonic – characterised by marked motor abnormalities including immobility.

Chloasma – a skin condition in which brown patches occur primarily on the cheekbones, forehead and upper lip. It also may develop on the nose, chin, lower cheeks and sides of the neck. The dark patches usually have distinct edges. Chloasma is seen most frequently in young women taking birth control pills and also occurs commonly during pregnancy. It may develop in association with menopause, hormonal imbalance and ovarian disorders.

Cicatrisation – contraction of fibrous tissue, formed at a wound site by fibroblasts, reducing the size of the wound but causing tissue distortion and disfigurement.

Circinate – circular; ring-shaped.

Commensal – living in a relationship in which one organism derives food or other benefits from another organism without hurting or helping it.

Coronal sulcus – the 'groove' behind the corona at the back of the glans. The flared rim at the back of the glans. This is the most sensitive part of the penis.

Crohn's disease – Crohn's disease causes inflammation in the small intestine. Crohn's disease usually occurs in the lower part of the small intestine, called the ileum, but it can affect any part of the digestive tract, from the mouth to the anus. The inflammation extends deep into the lining of the affected organ. The inflammation can cause pain and can make the intestines empty frequently, resulting in diarrhoea.

Cyst – a cyst is a fluid-filled sac, and can be located anywhere in the body.

Disulfiram – a carbamate derivative used as an alcohol deterrent. It is a relatively non-toxic substance when administered alone, but markedly alters the intermediary metabolism of alcohol. When alcohol is ingested after administration of disulfiram, blood acetaldehyde concentrations are increased, followed by flushing, systemic vasodilation, respiratory difficulties, nausea, hypotension, and other symptoms (acetaldehyde syndrome). The intensity and duration of symptoms vary greatly from individual to individual.

Dysaesthesia – impairment of any of the senses, especially of touch.

Dyscrasia – a term formerly used to indicate an abnormal mixture of the four humours; in surviving usages it now is roughly synonymous with disease or pathologic condition.

Dysmenorrhoea – painful menstruation.

Dyspareunia – deep lower abdominal pain.

Dysplasia – abnormality of development. In pathology: alteration in size, shape and organisation of adult cells.

Dysuria – difficult or painful discharge of urine.

Ectropian – this describes the situation in which columnar epithelium, continuous with that of the cervical canal, replaces the stratified squamous epithelium that normally covers the vaginal portion of the cervix.

EIA – enzyme immuno-assay (aka: ELISA), a specific treponemal antibody test for syphilis.

ELISA – the enzyme-linked immunosorbent assay is a serologic test used as a general screening tool for the detection of antibodies to the HIV virus. Reported as positive or negative. ELISA technology links a measurable enzyme to either an antigen or antibody. In this way, it can then measure the presence of an antibody or an antigen in the bloodstream.

Ergot – a disease of cereal plants (rye, wheat, etc.) caused by the fungus *Claviceps purpurea*; this fungus produces toxic alkaloids that, if ingested, cause symptoms such as hallucinations, severe gastrointestinal upset, a burning sensation in the limbs and extremities (St Anthony's Fire) and a form of gangrene.

ESR (erythrocyte sedimentation rate) – a test that measures the rate at which red blood cells settle through a column of liquid. A non-specific index of inflammation.

Exophytic – denoting a neoplasm or lesion that grows outward from an epithelial surface.

Fibroids – a benign tumour, especially of the uterine wall, that consists of fibrous and muscular tissue.

Flaviviridae – a family of single-stranded RNA-containing viruses that cause haemorrhagic fever in a wide range of mammals and are transmitted by mosquitos and ticks.

Fluorescent treponemal antibody-absorption, FTA-ABS – this test for syphilis is a blood serum screening test designed to demonstrate the presence or absence of specific antibodies directed against the organism (*Treponema pallidum*) responsible for syphilis. The test detects the majority but not all cases of the disease. It is thus a way of screening for the disease.

Fornix – an anatomical arch or fold: as the vaulted upper part of the vagina surrounding the uterine cervix.

Haemolytic – destructive to blood cells, resulting in liberation of haemoglobin.

Hepadna – a family of DNA-containing viruses that cause hepatitis in a wide range of vertebrate species.

Hypoplasia – the incomplete development or underdevelopment of an organ or tissue.

Icteric – relating to or marked by jaundice.

Imidazole – a five-membered heterocyclic compound occurring in l-histidine and other biologically important compounds.

Intrathecal – within a sheath; for example, cerebrospinal fluid that is contained within the dura mater. It also refers to drugs administered into the cerebrospinal fluid bathing the spinal cord and brain.

In vitro – within a glass, observable in a test tube, in an artificial environment.

In vivo – within the living body.

Jarisch Herxheimer reaction – an inflammatory reaction in syphilitic tissues (skin, mucous membrane, nervous system, or viscera) induced in certain cases by specific treatment with Salvarsan, mercury or antibiotics; believed to be due to a rapid release of treponemal antigen with an associated allergic reaction in the patient.

Lactam – one of a series of anhydrides of an amido type, analogous to the lactones, as oxindol.

Laparoscopy – 1: visual examination of the inside of the abdomen by means of a laparoscope (called also *peritoneoscopy*)
2: an operation (as tubal ligation or gallbladder removal) involving laparoscopy.

Laparotomy – surgical section of the abdominal wall.

LFT – liver function test.

Lithotomy – the operation, art or practice of cutting for stone in the bladder.

Lupus erythematosus – systemic lupus erythematosus (SLE) is a disease of the immune system (the system that prevents and fights infection). In lupus the immune system becomes unbalanced, resulting in the body reacting against healthy tissue. This is why the symptoms of lupus can vary so much. Occasionally the disease is caused by using certain drugs. This is known as drug-induced lupus. SLE is classified as a rheumatic disease. It can cause inflammation in the joints and several of the body's organ systems. (For example: the skin, the kidneys and various other internal organs.) Hence the term 'systemic'. The term 'lupus erythematosus' refers to the red rash on the face. Discoid lupus affects the skin and is a relatively mild disease. Sometimes it is treated by a rheumatologist (a specialist in arthritis and rheumatic disease) but more commonly by a dermatologist (a specialist in skin disorders).

Lymphangitis – inflammation of a lymphatic vessel or vessels. Acute lymphangitis may result from spread of bacterial infection (most commonly beta haemolytic streptococci) into the lymphatics, manifested by painful subcutaneous red streaks along the course of the vessels.

Macrolide – a group of antibiotics produced by various strains of Streptomyces that have a complex macrocyclic structure. They inhibit protein synthesis by blocking the 50S ribosomal subunit. Include erythromycin, carbomycin. Used clinically as broad-spectrum antibiotics, particularly against Gram-positive bacteria.

Macroscopic – items large enough to be observed by the naked eye.

Macule – a spot, only commonly met in the construct 'immaculate' meaning unspotted.

Menorrhagia – abnormally profuse menstrual flow.

Mittlesmirch – pain with ovulation.

Moiety – originally, a half; now, loosely, a portion of something, Functional group.

Mordant – any substance, as alum or copperas, which, having a twofold attraction for organic fibres and colouring matter, serves as a bond of union, and thus gives fixity to, or bites in, the dyes.

Multivalent – having a valence greater than one, the number of binding sites on a molecule.

Myalgia – pain in a muscle or muscles.

Nabothian cyst – a Nabothian cyst is a mucus-filled cyst on the surface of the uterine cervix.

Nulliparous – of, relating to, or being a female that has not borne offspring.

Parabens – proprietary name for the methyl, propyl, butyl and ethyl esters of p-hydroxybenzoic acid. They have been approved by the FDA as antimicrobial agents for foods and pharmaceuticals.

Paraesthesia – morbid or perverted sensation, an abnormal sensation, as burning, prickling, formication, etc.

Parametritis – inflammation of the cellular tissue in the vicinity of the uterus.

Parous – having produced offspring.

Parturition – the act or process of giving birth to a child.

Pathognomonic – specially or decisively characteristic of a disease.

Pedunculated – the stalk of an inflorescence; in ferns, the stalk of a sporocarp.

Picorna – a family of single-stranded RNA-containing viruses that cause hepatitis in humans.

Polyene – a chemical compound having a series of conjugated (alternating) double bonds; e.g. the carotenoids.

Porphyria – a pathological state in man and some lower animals that is often due to genetic factors, is characterised by abnormalities of porphyrin metabolism and results in the excretion of large quantities of porphyrins in the urine and in extreme sensitivity to light. Porphyrins are pigments found in both animal and plant life.

Proctitis – inflammation of the rectum.

Proctoscopy – endoscopic examination of the rectum.

Prodromal – an early or premonitory symptom of a disease.

Prozone reaction – antibody excess.

Pruritis – itching.

PT – prothrombin time.

Puerperal – of or pertaining to childbirth.

Pyrethrin – a substance resembling, and isomeric with, ordinary camphor, and extracted from the essential oil of feverfew.

Pyrethroid – synthetic pyrethrin derivatives that are used as insecticides; as a class these agents are less toxic to mammals than are other effective insecticides.

Radiculopathy – a herniated intervertebral disk (nucleus pulposus) is one which has become displaced (prolapsed) from its normal position in between the vertebral bodies of the spine.

Refractory – not readily yielding to treatment.

Retinoid – derivatives of vitamin A. Used clinically in the treatment of severe cystic acne, psoriasis, and other disorders of keratinisation.

Rimming – licking someone's anus.

RPR test – rapid plasma reagin, a common non-specific treponemal antibody test.

Salicylates – the salts, esters of salicylic acids, or salicylate esters of an organic acid. Some of these have analgesic, antipyretic and anti-inflammatory activities by inhibiting prostaglandin synthesis.

Sarcoidosis – a multisystem disorder characterised in affected organs by a type of inflammation called granulomas. The cause is unknown.

Schlerosis – a medical condition which causes a hardening of body tissue or organs, especially the arteries.

Scotoma – an area of lost or depressed vision within the visual field, surrounded by an area of less depressed or of normal vision.

Septate vagina – a vagina that is divided, usually longitudinally, to create a double vagina.

Serovars – a subdivision of a species or subspecies distinguishable from other strains therein on the basis of antigenic character. Synonym: serotype.

Sinus – a notch, depression or cavity on the surface of an organ.

Spirochaetes – an elongated, spirally shaped bacterium, for example the organism responsible for syphilis.

Tendonitis – inflammation of the tendons.

Torsades de pointes – a cardiac arrhythmia, which may cause blackouts or even sudden death. The phrase 'torsades de pointes' is French and literally means 'twisting of the points', referring to the characteristic appearance of the electrocardiogram during the rhythm abnormality. Torsades de pointes usually occurs in the setting of a prolonged QT interval on the electrocardiogram. Torsades de pointes occurs in individuals with genetic mutations in genes that control expression of sodium or potassium channels and is a frequent cause of sudden death in these individuals. It also occurs as a complication of drugs that prolong the QT interval by blockade of potassium channels.

Toxic shock syndrome – a blood-borne bacterial infection caused by the genus *Staphylococcus*. Usually affects menstruating females under the age of 30 and was associated in the past with the use of a particular type of tampon (no longer used).

Tpha – *Treponema pallidum* haemagglutination assay is a highly specific test for treponema antigens.

Treponeme – a vernacular term used to refer to any member of the genus *Treponema*. Genus of bacteria of the spirochaete family (*Spirochaetaceae*). *Treponema pallidum* causes syphilis. Cells are corkscrew-like, motile, anaerobic and with a peptidoglycan cell wall and a capsule of glycosaminoglycans similar to hyaluronic acid and chondroitin sulphate in composition. Membrane has cardiolipin.

Ulcerative colitis – a disease that causes inflammation and sores, called ulcers, in the lining of the large intestine. The inflammation usually occurs in the rectum and lower part of the colon, but it may affect the entire colon.

Vaginismus – a painful spasmodic contraction of the vagina, often rendering copulation impossible.

VDRL – Venereal Disease Research Laboratory.

Venous thromboembolism (sometimes called thrombophlebitis) – a term used to describe a blood clot in a vein, which often becomes painful, red and swollen. When a blood clot forms in a vein it may partially or completely block the flow of blood in that vein. If this occurs in one of the deep veins in the body it is called a deep venous thrombosis (DVT). The most common sites for blood clots to form are the legs and pelvis, but it can also occur in the arms.

Wilson's disease – a genetic disorder that is fatal unless detected and treated before serious illness from copper poisoning develops. The genetic defect causes excessive copper accumulation in the liver or brain. Excess copper attacks the liver or brain, resulting in hepatitis, psychiatric or neurologic symptoms.

Reference

1 Amsel RP, Totten CA, Spiegel KC *et al.* (1983) Nonspecific vaginitis: diagnostic criteria and microbial and epidemiologic associations. *American Journal of Medicine.* **74**: 14–22.

Index

Page numbers in *italic* refer to tables or figures.